Power Source
for Women

SUSAN SOMMERS   THERESA DUGWELL

Power Source for Women

Proven Fitness Strategies, Tools, and Success Stories for Women 45+

Toronto and New York
bpsbooks.com

Published in 2010 by
BPS Books
Toronto and New York
www.bpsbooks.com
A division of Bastian Publishing Services Ltd.

ISBN 978-1-926645-20-9
Cataloguing-in-Publication Data available from Library and Archives Canada.

Cover: Gnibel
Text design and typesetting: Casey Hooper Design
Photographs: Shahrokh Saeedi
Line drawings: Heidi Overhill

Printed by Lightning Source, Tennessee. Lightning Source paper, as used in this book, does not come from endangered old growth forests or forests of exceptional conservation value. It is acid free, lignin free, and meets all ANSI standards for archival-quality paper. The print-on-demand used to produce this book protects the environment by printing only the number of copies that are purchased.

This book is dedicated to our mothers:

Lee Sommers,
for encouraging me, believing in me, and inspiring me.
In my mind and my heart, you will always be
my role model and my power source.

Margaret Ayer,
for having the courage to change, the wisdom to find your inner peace,
and the strength for motherhood. You have become my inspiration,
my advisor, and my confidante. Thank you for all the ways
you have helped me to grow — Mother, I love you so.

Contents

PART 1 / MENTAL FITNESS: CHANGE YOUR MIND

Power Source Tool #1

Power Source Tool #2

PART 3 / EMOTIONAL FITNESS: CHANGE YOUR LIFE

Power Source Tool #8

RECOGNIZE CHALLENGES, PERSEVERE, AND
REFOCUS ON YOUR FITNESS GOALS

Power Source Tool #9

CREATE REWARDS AND CELEBRATE YOUR SUCCESSES

Preface

Power Source for Women is dedicated to women 45+ at all levels, stages, and abilities of fitness. Our simple, realistic approach touches on the very essence of what we can do as women to develop a healthy body, mind, and spirit. Throughout this book we provide specific, research-based strategies and tools that are especially appropriate for women.

We are committed to your fitness. We have written *Power Source for Women* to help get you started and to help keep you motivated, by showing you the amazing rewards that come from fitness. We will help you to launch your fitness journey and to persevere one step at a time. We will show you how you can be a mentor and inspiration to other women and girls. In our approach, as you will see, the richest and most lasting rewards are in the journey, not the destination.

You may be wondering how we became so inspired by fitness.

Susan's Story

Growing up in the suburbs of New Jersey, I was introduced to a number of sports. My father taught my older brother, Howard, and me how to roller skate, ice skate, swim, and ride a bike when we were young.

I now realize that my father was at the forefront of the home gym movement. In the 1950s he set up a rowing machine, a chinning bar, and hand weights in the basement of our house. My brother, who was recovering from polio, exercised with him. However, as a girl in that traditional decade, I was not encouraged to try the machines and the weights. In fact, it took me another 40 years to get involved in strength training.

I was always quite short and loved candy and cookies. From the time I was 10 until I started to smoke at the age of 16, I was self-conscious about my weight. For the next 20 years, I controlled it through a combination of smoking, dieting, and diet pills.

My mother and her two sisters were also obsessed with weight — their own and that of their three daughters. When I went away to university, I took a black coat with me: Whenever I gained weight, I wore it for when I was getting off the plane to meet my mother.

When I stopped smoking in 1980, I gained 25 pounds. For the next 15 years, I tried to lose the weight through aerobics classes, swimming, skipping meals, and all kinds of diets — with little success.

THE TURNING POINT

As I entered my 50s and menopause, I knew I had to change my eating habits, find healthier tools for dealing with stress, and discover new ways to relax.

When I started to work full-time at a YMCA Business Centre near Toronto in 2002, I received two free YMCA fitness memberships — one for me and one for my husband, Peter. At the age of 57 I joined a Saturday YMCA Run Fit class and started to jog.

Jogging, walking, and weight training became my passion. From 2002 to 2010 I trained for, and completed, ten 5k runs, three 10ks, 10 half-marathons, and two full marathons.

During that time I also watched my mother fight chronic

pain due to osteoarthritis and gradually lose her mobility. When she died in early 2009 from Alzheimer's disease, she was bedridden. This gave me an added incentive to keep moving. I vowed I would increase my core strength and flexibility through a more disciplined fitness program.

Today I am 20 pounds lighter, and, through weight training and walking/jogging, I have totally transformed my body. I am proud of the way I look and now realize *this is* the best me.

Theresa's Story

My childhood was challenged by the absence of my father and the presence of a young mother who suffered from bouts of depression and anxiety. I recall the many nights I consoled her and the many times I wished for a better life — one with a mother who could nurture me emotionally and a father figure to guide and protect me. My two siblings, both younger than I, on many occasions looked to me for parental leadership throughout our childhood years.

THE TURNING POINT

The challenges I faced as a young girl certainly increased my susceptibility to depression, and not having strong parental guidance during difficult times put me at emotional risk. What kept me motivated and free from depression and adolescent turmoil was the occasional quiet voice within reminding me that one day I would grow up and my life could change.

It was painful and exhausting at times for me to watch my mother suffer in her emotionally distraught world and to try so desperately to help her.

Looking at this in a positive light, I see that these early experiences prompted me to take a keen interest in understanding how to build a stronger mind and body. As an adolescent I found escaping to my bedroom, closing the door, listening to music, and exercising to be a great way to put myself in a better state. As I entered adulthood I continued to use exercise and nutrition as my formula for looking and feeling better. Today I have a lifelong commitment to physical fitness and my well-being.

As a result of my early exposure to my mother's emotional challenges, I have become a more resilient person, with greater adaptability and flexibility in challenging situations. I have developed a good stress-management system and I strive to keep a positive mindset and have a good attitude each day. I also recognize that my healthy lifestyle and regular physical exercise together make up the major contributing factor to my level of daily optimal functioning — my survival tool; the key to my being the best I can be.

As I look back I recognize that during those early years my mother did not have the mindset she needed to make changes. She did not have a support system, she did not have the knowledge, and she did not have the power source from within to feel confident enough to search for ways to change. I was too young to make a difference in her life; all I could do at the time was be there to comfort her when the world seemed so lonely. Those were important times because they helped build two things for me: a curiosity to understand my mother's challenges and a determination to become the best I could be, both physically and mentally.

I am pleased to say that today my mother has conquered that internal demon called depression and she is a revitalized woman. She has a strong support system and has the necessary structure and warmth in her life to keep her in a positive light. Recently my mother decided to make physical fitness a part of her healthy lifestyle and has joined me at the YMCA. I am proud of the woman she has become and grateful for all she has taught me about life. Today she is the mother I always hoped for. Through her I have learned it is never too late to change when you find the power source within.

Our Story Together

We met in the summer of 2007 at a Toronto YMCA, where we were both members. We talked about all of the wonderful, inspiring women — from 22 to 90 years of age — we saw working out at six in the morning and how they could motivate other women to commit to fitness.

The women included those in excellent health and those who were dealing with a variety of problems and issues, such as poor eyesight, multiple sclerosis, cancer, and arthritis. We realized these women had stories to tell.

In the fall of 2007 the YMCA Women's Workshop Series "Celebrating Our Y Women" was created to give these and other women an opportunity to develop their stories into a presentation, assisted by Theresa. The purpose of the workshops designed from the stories was to educate, inspire, motivate, and build community. The wonderful outcome of this experience was that the women found a power source from within and were eager to do more.

One of us, Susan, was the first speaker, in October 2007, shortly after completing her second marathon at the age of 63. Subsequently, eight other women were invited to tell their stories and to share their successes and challenges. In fact, some of the women you will meet in this book — Gloria Jacobs, Claire Vandramini, Abbey Smith, and Edna Levitt — appeared as speakers in this workshop series.

The series was an overwhelming success. As other women heard about the events, they contacted us for advice and inspiration. As a result, we decided in the fall of 2009 to write a book composed of fitness strategies, tools, and success stories for women 45+.

We set a number of goals for this book, as well as for our speaking engagements, coaching, and website.

These include to:

- encourage women to embrace their strengths, passions, gifts, and successes
- show women how they can invent, and live, their best lives through their commitment to fitness
- motivate women to make decisions for lifelong health and vitality
- promote disease prevention through fitness
- use humor and personal stories to motivate women to take action
- showcase role models who would inspire other women and girls, share their success stories, and offer fitness advice
- provide women with self-assessment tools, quizzes, and questionnaires, as well as opportunities to find the FIT relationship that is most compatible with their lives
- create the North York YMCA Women's Fund, a program that assists women in shelters who are survivors of violence and abuse[*]
- develop an online community, through our new website and blog www.powersourceforwomen.com, for women to connect with other women, share their stories, download information, and build their own accountability teams and fitness network.

Chief among these goals was writing *Power Source for Women* and getting it into the hands of people just like you. We hope you will find your source of energy and wisdom from reading this book and will take advantage of the Power Source approach to your mental, physical, and emotional fitness.

Susan Sommers
Theresa Dugwell

---

[*] This program provides YMCA memberships to women during a critical life-transition, giving them access to a place of community, health, and support for personal growth. A portion of the proceeds from book sales and other product sales will be donated to this fund.

Introduction

Today more than ever before, women are running, spinning, cycling, golfing, skiing, dancing, weight-training, swimming, walking, and, of course, practicing yoga and Pilates. Yet there are surprisingly few resources on fitness for women.

Consider this book — and its associated website www.powersourceforwomen.com — your place to meet other women who will inspire and support you in your lifelong journey to fitness.

HEALTH ISSUES FOR WOMEN 45+

Today's women 45+ are saucier, bolder, more youthful, and more outspoken than ever before. Yet, as women age, they often experience a number of health problems and chronic conditions, such as back problems, arthritis, rheumatism, heart disease, vision problems, high blood pressure, and hearing loss. This book's advice, should any of these things happen to you, is to acknowledge your frustrations *and* commit to living life as fully as possible. There are so many ways to stay active, no matter what your age or stage, and no matter what your fitness needs and physical abilities.

You can create a fitness program that is appropriate for *your* body, mind, and spirit.

FOUR TRENDS IN FITNESS

Our approach to mental, physical, and emotional fitness picks up on four major trends in the world of fitness today. These are Green Fitness, Daily Fitness, Functional Training, and Accountability Teams.

GREEN FITNESS

Throughout this book we highlight a number of Green FIT ways for you to incorporate physical fitness *and* care for the environment into your program of exercise and physical activities. You will see this symbol ⊛ in these parts of the book. These include:

- exercising outdoors, including regular walking, hiking, swimming, running, yoga, and bike riding
- planting a vegetable garden or an herb garden — and eating fresh from your garden
- buying your produce from a co-op or a local farmers' market
- eating lean and organic meats
- buying recycled or slightly worn workout clothes and equipment
- making your own weights from household objects
- taking Green FIT vacations.

DAILY FITNESS

It is more and more accepted by medical experts and the public that some type of physical activity or regular exercise *daily* is essential for long-term fitness and health. Research shows that taking part in activities throughout the day that keep you moving for a total of 30 to 60 minutes can greatly benefit your health and well-being.

Simply adding movement into your daily routine can increase your level of fitness. For example, you can park in the last row of the parking lot and walk between your office and your car. You can walk up and down the stairs, get off the bus or subway several stops early and walk the extra distance, walk the dog for 10 minutes when you get home, go mall walking, ride a bicycle, garden, mow the lawn, or shovel snow.

FUNCTIONAL TRAINING

Functional fitness involves doing exercises that will enable you to perform daily activities more effectively. For those of you who are baby boomers, these exercises are crucial tools for preventing injury as you age.

Whatever your age, you can create a functional fitness program with exercises that rely on your body weight to increase your strength. Functional training includes pushing your children or grandchildren on the swings, vacuuming, working in the garden, raking leaves, carrying groceries, opening jars, climbing stairs, lifting a suitcase, carrying a child, squatting to tie a shoelace without feeling pain, or standing on tiptoe to reach something on the top shelf.

Functional training exercises require balance, coordination, and stability. These exercises can be more challenging than traditional strength training, which uses machines to support your body weight. Some of the exercises included in functional fitness are squats, overhead reaches, rowing motions, and forward presses.

In the chapter *Power Source Tool #7*, we offer you our own Functional FIT Workout Plan; this workout takes only 20 to 30 minutes to complete. (See pages 121–26.)

ACCOUNTABILITY TEAMS

Research shows that becoming part of a group or team that holds them accountable to change is a particularly important ingredient in fitness success for women.

Throughout the book, we encourage you to build a network of people who will support you and keep you motivated in your fitness commitment. Keep in touch with them on a daily or weekly basis in person, by phone, through e-mail, on Facebook, or through Twitter. Your accountability team will sustain you through any setbacks you experience, encourage you to fulfill your dreams, and celebrate with you as you succeed along the way.

NO MORE EXCUSES

You know the importance of getting in shape, but you also know the time and effort it requires. You may feel you don't have enough time to exercise. When it's time to actually get out there and start to move, many women have a long list of reasons not to exercise. We've heard them all (and used some of them ourselves):

- ✓ I'm too busy
- ✓ I'm too tired.
- ✓ I don't have time.
- ✓ I'll never look like (insert a celeb name of your choice), so why bother?
- ✓ I can't afford the expensive equipment or the health club membership I need to get fit.
- ✓ Exercise is boring.
- ✓ I have arthritis or stiff joints.
- ✓ I don't like to work out.
- ✓ I'm too sore from my last workout.
- ✓ I'm getting sick.
- ✓ I feel guilty about taking the time for myself.
- ✓ I am unsteady on my feet; I'm afraid of falling.
- ✓ I have concerns about my heart.
- ✓ My friends and family don't support my efforts to work out.
- ✓ I'm too lazy.
- ✓ I'm self-conscious about how I look when I exercise.
- ✓ I'm not athletic.
- ✓ I'm intimidated by the young instructors.
- ✓ I always quit.
- ✓ I'm too stressed.
- ✓ It's too cold.

✓ It's too dark.

✓ It will be too difficult.

✓ I can't allow myself to fail.

✓ I can't change.

✓ I'm too old.

The issue is how you're going to get beyond the excuses and start to move. *Power Source for Women* will provide you with a step-by-step guide to getting past the negativity and securely on your way to fitness success.

WHAT WE COVER

Power Source for Women is divided into three parts, dealing first with mental fitness (because everything starts with your outlook), then with physical fitness, and then with emotional fitness (which is intimately linked to being physically fit). Each part is composed of chapters that share not only our own story but also the wisdom of three groups of women: our Power Source Experts, Power Source Role Models, and Power Source Women (see pages 9–12 below).

As you progress through the book, you will be inspired to change your mind, change your body, and change your emotions. We take you chapter by chapter through the process of identifying your needs, building an accountability team, defining what success is for you, setting personal goals, and creating fitness routines that fit your goals.

We also help you discover your FIT Motivational Style™, create your FIT Action Plan, and develop ways to celebrate your success and set new goals.

NO TIME LIKE THE PRESENT

As women, each day we get up and go about our normal routines. These usually involve many responsibilities, from caring for a family or aging parent(s) to working outside the home in order to earn a living for our family and ourselves. Sometimes we're so consumed by life's demands, we don't notice that we're not nurturing ourselves mentally, physically, and emotionally.

It's time for you to delve deeper into your life and evaluate what you are currently doing for yourself. Ask yourself two questions: Who am I (independent of my family, friends, work, and responsibilities)? How am I taking care of myself?

There's no time like the present to begin to nurture yourself. Take the opportunity, as you travel through this book, to think beyond where you are today. Take the time to learn about yourself and to explore the information you find here. Travel through this book with an open mind and be inspired. You have one life and if you aren't feeling great right now, it's time for a change. It's true that a deep sense of satisfaction can come from caring for others and ensuring that their needs are met. But remember, time does not stand still. Start to nurture *yourself* today. Tap into your capacity for greatness.

THE TRUE MEANING OF A HEALTHY LIFESTYLE

The World Health Organization (WHO) states that "health is a state of complete physical, mental, and social well-being." Health is not defined as simply the absence of disease. According to WHO, "The actual definition of Healthy Living is the steps, actions and strategies one puts in place to achieve optimum health." Living a healthy lifestyle requires that you take responsibility and make smarter choices today and in your future.

ACHIEVING A HEALTHY LIFESTYLE

So how do you achieve a healthy lifestyle? Does it mean you should never eat cake or drink a glass of wine? Or that you have to exercise every day and make sure you get eight hours of sleep every night?

When your lifestyle has involved poor eating habits, a lack of sleep, or relationship problems, or if you just don't have any time for yourself, making changes can seem overwhelming. But creating a healthy lifestyle doesn't mean you have to make drastic changes all at once. In fact, drastic changes can be more difficult to stick with. Making small changes in the way you live each day can lead to big rewards. Remember, you have taken the first step to making changes: recognizing that your current ways are incongruent with the way you want to live.

CREATE YOUR OWN POWER SOURCE STORY

Over the years, we have achieved many fitness goals and encountered many obstacles and setbacks, and yet we continue to set new, challenging goals. We believe our experiences will help you as you set and reach your fitness goals. That's why we share our stories with you at the beginning of each chapter.

Another feature of this book is its emphasis on journaling as a way to grow into fitness. At the end of each chapter, journaling expert Lesley Shore encourages you to create your own FIT Journal. Her insights, thought-provoking questions, and emotional support will help you to get started on what can become a lifetime practice.

In addition, we encourage *you* to send us *your* stories, successes, and challenges. We'd love to hear from you. You can reach us online by going to www.powersourceforwomen.com. Through this online meeting place and through our speaking and consulting, we are building a community of women who are developing a safe place, an inspiring and empowering place, a place from which they can reach out to other women in need.

We hope you enjoy reading and using this book as much as we did writing it. Make fitness *your* passion and find your own power source within.

Meet Your Power Source Support Team

POWER SOURCE EXPERTS

We invited two outstanding women, Ruth Krongold and Lesley Shore, to be the experts on our Power Source team. Their full biographies are included at the end of this book. We'll just introduce them to you here.

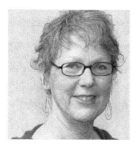

Ruth Krongold, BA, MSW, RSW,
Psychotherapy and Family Mediation, 59

Ruth is our Power Source Emotional Fitness Expert. She is an experienced counselor, facilitator, and family mediator with individual, relationship, family, and group psychotherapy expertise gained in a variety of community and private settings. Ruth now enjoys an independent practice. She assists adults and children who want to find constructive alternatives that diminish the effects of their problems and amplify hopeful outcomes.

Ruth currently swims about 2 miles (3.25 kilometers) daily. While the YMCA pool is her usual spot for swimming, she prefers to be out of doors on lakes, rivers, seas, or oceans as the opportunity arises. She conservatively estimates that she swims about 60 miles (100 kilometers) per year and has done so for more than three decades. As well, she participates in aqua fit classes and loves to hike, canoe, kayak, snowshoe, and cross-country ski when the conditions are right.

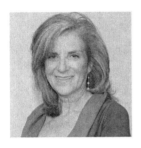

Lesley Z. Shore, EdD, 63

Lesley, our Power Source Journaling Expert, was Assistant Professor in the Department of Curriculum, Teaching and Learning, responsible for Intermediate/Secondary English at the Ontario Institute for Studies in Education (OISE), University of Toronto.

In her course Anne Frank and the Writing of the Adolescent Self, Lesley honored the importance of journal writing in the development of identity. Writers and writing are her passion. Lesley has been journaling since she was 14 years old.

POWER SOURCE ROLE MODELS

We selected five women to feature in our book as our Role Models — women who have overcome adversity and achieved goals most women would only dare to dream about: Claire Vandramini, Maureen Catania, Abbey Smith, Gloria Jacobs, and Sheila Rhodes. These women's achievements have transformed their lives and given them the tools for ongoing success in physical, mental, and emotional fitness. Their achievements have encouraged them to develop a passion for fitness and a healthy body and mind and to mentor other women.

We asked these women to share their triumphs and challenges on their way to fitness success and to explain what they do to stay committed, motivated, and strong. They share their stories and fitness experiences throughout the book with hope, humor, and inspiration.

Claire Vandramini, 63

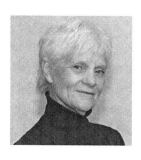

Claire started cycling 11 years ago to get a little relief from the stress and hurt she felt when her husband was undergoing his many cancer treatments. As a result of this decision, she later found that her love of cycling and fitness took on a whole new meaning. In July 2009 Claire completed her first Ironman 70.3 in Peterborough, Ontario (Canada), and finished second in her age category. In September of the same year, she traveled to Australia to compete in the World Olympic Triathlon. In April 2010 she competed in Galveston, Texas, and qualified for the 2010 World Ironman 70.3 Championships in Tampa, Florida. To date she has enjoyed many different triathlons, both long and short. Her goal in 2011 is to complete in her first full Ironman and get her "finisher" Ironman tattoo.

Maureen Catania, 50

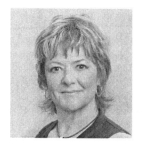

Over a period of three years, Maureen lost 50 inches and 50 pounds. Her daily fitness program involves a combination of strength training and weights. She has replaced her entire wardrobe and is now wearing sexy dresses and heels.

Abbey Smith, 69

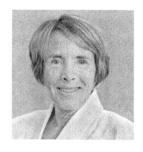

In her 50s, when her adolescent daughter told her there was "nothing she could do" to keep her off the streets at night, Abbey enrolled them both in a women's self-defense class where they practiced awareness, alertness, and defensive actions. It was there that Abbey first heard about Aikido. At the age of 67, after 12 years of training, Abbey received her first-degree black belt in Aikido (Shodan). The oldest female member of the Shugyo Dojo Toronto, Abbey teaches Aikido to children and adults and continues to train.

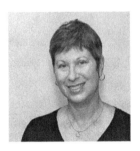

Gloria Jacobs, 59

For the past seven years, Gloria has been a member of Dragon Boat Racing teams. In the summer of 2005 she participated at the World Dragon Boat Competition in Berlin. In April 2007, while training on the Canadian team for the World Dragon Boat in Australia, Gloria discovered she had breast cancer. She had a lumpectomy, underwent radiation, and continued to train. Her team won a silver medal and a bronze medal.

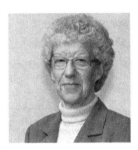

Sheila Rhodes, 59

A fitness educator and a lifelong athlete committed to a healthy lifestyle, Sheila underwent emergency quadruple by-pass surgery in 2003. She recovered fully through a combination of cycle fit, weight training, running, and yoga.

POWER SOURCE WOMEN

Since the fall of 2007, we have talked to hundreds of women from 45 to 90 years of age about their lives and their relationships with fitness. We've invited six of these women to be part of our book: Audrey Korey, Edna Levitt, Pat McMonagle, Phyllis Naken, Monika Klein, and Dorina Vendramin. They represent women everywhere who continue to astound us, delight us, and inspire us by what they achieve with their minds and bodies. These women provide insights throughout *Power Source for Women* — insights into their own fitness successes, challenges, obstacles, and dreams. Their biographies are included at the end of the book.

Getting Started

We hope you will take this opportunity, before you get into the content of this book, to test yourself on the myths and facts of fitness and healthy living. You can do this by:

- taking our FIT Savvy Quiz™
- completing our FIT Lifestyle Questionnaire™
- reviewing some tips for healthy living.

TAKE OUR FIT SAVVY QUIZ™

This quiz will help you see how and why physical activity and a physical lifestyle are critical for increasing your daily level of functioning and for helping you live a longer, happier life. Rev up your mind as you think through your answers to the following questions about fitness (you may already be asking yourself some of them).

1. Natural athletic ability is a prerequisite to physical activity.
True
False

2. Creating a healthy lifestyle doesn't mean you have to make drastic changes all at once.
True
False

3. Surrounding yourself with people who exercise regularly can help you stick to your program of fitness.
True
False

4. Your level of motivation will not make or break your fitness program.
True
False

5. Intrinsic motivation is striving inwardly to be good at something and to reward yourself inwardly for your successes.
True
False

6. When sticking to a fitness program and beginning to see results, public verbal recognition from friends and family telling you how great you look or asking if you've lost weight will help you as a form of intrinsic motivation.
True
False

7. New activities, such as square dancing, tai chi, and yoga, engage your brain and challenge it; this process is similar to the way physical activity engages your body.
True
False

8. Adults who spend time each day engaging in physical activity reduce risk factors associated with aging, as well as add years to their lives.
True
False

9. Exercise doesn't affect your sleep.
True
False

10. Walking each day can help you build and strengthen muscle mass.
True
False

ANSWERS TO OUR FIT SAVVY QUIZ™

1. False
Natural athletic ability is not a prerequisite to physical activity. Simply focus on the positive changes you are making to your body and mind.

2. True
Drastic changes can be more difficult to stick with. Making small changes in how you live each day can lead to big rewards.

3. True
Studies show that people who take classes with other people, join a team, connect through e-mail and online coaching, or work out with other people have the highest fitness success rates.

4. False
Motivation is possibly the biggest determining factor when it comes to creating and implementing a fitness program.

5. True
When the activity is experienced as rewarding in and of itself, there is little need for external motivators to get you activated. Intrinsic motivation can come from love of a particular activity, self-satisfaction, and a sense of achievement and purpose.

6. False
This is an extrinsic motivator, also known as an outside reward. These types of rewards provide satisfaction and pleasure, but they do not increase your internal motivation as you try to build your fitness program. That said, they can still play the important role of keeping you in the game.

7. True

Consider your brain a muscle and find ways to engage it just like your physical body. Keeping your mind active with new experiences and exercise is just as important as working out.

8. True

By engaging in daily physical activity you can reduce your risk of chronic diseases, such as heart disease, high blood pressure, and osteoporosis. You will also experience increased psychological well-being and reduced feelings of depression and anxiety.

9. False

Exercise can make your sleep deeper, meaning it will be more refreshing and you will rest more peacefully throughout the night.

10. True

However, the building of muscles through walking will depend on the intensity of the walk. It needs to be a brisk walk and include variations. Using light wrist weights, for example, will help you to target the toning of your arms.

COMPLETE OUR FIT LIFESTYLE QUESTIONNAIRE™

The following FIT Lifestyle Questionnaire™ is a self-assessment tool to help you see how you measure up to the elements that represent a healthy lifestyle. Find out which FIT Lifestyle level best reflects your current values and attitudes toward health and fitness. Throughout this book we suggest FIT lifestyle habits that will help you to gain a healthier body and mind, develop better stress management tools, and find the motivation to reach your goals.

Be honest when you make your selections and choose only one response. You'll have a chance after you take the questionnaire to add up your responses and get feedback on your results.

Today is the first day on your journey to positive lifestyle changes. Don't be discouraged by where you are right now. You are on your way to a healthier body and lifestyle.

THE FIT LIFESTYLE QUESTIONNAIRE™

Select the FIT Lifestyle box for each question that best reflects how you are living TODAY. Be honest so you can clearly identify the areas where you need to achieve the greatest change.

	Never 0	Occa- sionally 1	Fre- quently 2	Always 3
I live by the motto: Early to bed, early to rise	❑	❑	❑	❑
I get 7–9 hours of sleep most nights	❑	❑	❑	❑
I have a good social network	❑	❑	❑	❑
I am grateful for the things in my life	❑	❑	❑	❑
I have a hobby I enjoy	❑	❑	❑	❑
I set goals for myself	❑	❑	❑	❑
I like to spend time with friends/family	❑	❑	❑	❑
I set aside time just for me	❑	❑	❑	❑
I enjoy my career/ work in or out of the home	❑	❑	❑	❑
I have a close friend/ partner with whom I can share my thoughts, goals, and frustrations	❑	❑	❑	❑
I like my body	❑	❑	❑	❑
I am happy	❑	❑	❑	❑
I exercise regularly	❑	❑	❑	❑

I enjoy outdoor activities	❏	❏	❏	❏
I have regular check-ups with my doctor	❏	❏	❏	❏
I reward myself when I reach a goal or for any achievement	❏	❏	❏	❏
Most of my meals are well-balanced and prepared in a healthy manner	❏	❏	❏	❏
I try to drink 6–8 glasses of water every day	❏	❏	❏	❏
I take short breaks during the day for myself	❏	❏	❏	❏
I enjoy reading or listening to health-related topics on self-improvement	❏	❏	❏	❏
I am good at problem solving	❏	❏	❏	❏
I am optimistic about my future	❏	❏	❏	❏
I eat healthy foods and occasionally reward myself with a treat	❏	❏	❏	❏
I have healthy ways to deal with my stress, such as meditation	❏	❏	❏	❏
I take action if I am dissatisfied with something in my life	❏	❏	❏	❏

8   34
      8
    42

CALCULATING YOUR FIT LIFESTYLE SCORE

SCORING PROCEDURE

Add up your points. (The point values are located above the four different response options.) Once you know your total, read below to see where you place on the FIT Lifestyle Scale and the course of action we suggest you consider to achieve your FIT Healthy Lifestyle.

FIT LIFESTYLE SCALE

| 5 | 10 | 15 | 20 | 25 | 30 | 35 | 40 | 45 | 5 0 | 55 | 60 | 65 | 70 | 75 |

Low 0–26   Average 27–53   Optimal 54–75

IF YOU SCORED 0–26 POINTS

It's time to take immediate action.

First of all, congratulations for completing this self-assessment questionnaire and especially for being honest. We believe you're reading this book because you really want to change things in your life and become healthier. You are probably feeling the negative effects of your lifestyle, both physically and mentally, on a daily basis. Your energy level may be very low, making it difficult for you to get motivated to make changes. We are ready to give you guidance through the strategies, tools, and success stories in this book.

But we suggest you visit your doctor first to discuss your current health status and your goals so you can move ahead on your journey to a better you. You want to make sure, as you travel through this book, that you can tap into all of the tools and start making changes. Get the go-ahead from your doctor and then start to move.

IF YOU SCORED 27–53 POINTS

Your lifestyle is okay, but it's time to make it better.

Your lifestyle could use some major changes. You have probably been feeling frustrated with yourself and somewhat stuck in a pattern you can't seem to change. Maybe it's all of the responsibilities that keep you on the move and give you little time to stop and think about your own needs.

Start by working on the aspects of your lifestyle where you answered "occasionally" and "never." You'll certainly discover the pay-off in your energy levels and sense of well-being by beginning with a few changes. Remember, one change at a time can add up quickly.

IF YOU SCORED 54–75 POINTS
Your lifestyle looks good. Why not make it great?

You are a shining example of someone who is trying to be proactive about your health, making choices that are good for you. You live a balanced lifestyle, but you may have a few areas you want to improve.

Well, here's your chance. Look over your responses and find the ones where you scored "occasionally" and "never." These are the areas that could use some attention. So get into action today and make the changes. You are probably already feeling great. So why not feel even better?

TIPS FOR HEALTHY LIVING

With your FIT Lifestyle Questionnaire™ results in hand, keep the following 16 healthy living tips in mind as you work toward building a healthier lifestyle.

1. Create balance by engaging in moderate behavior in your eating, working, resting, playing, hobbies, and socializing.
2. Take stock of how you spend your day. Concentrate on the important things that need to get done and cut down on the unnecessary items. This will help you to reduce your stress.
3. Learn how to say *no*. Don't take on too many things. This can sometimes lead to unnecessary stress and burnout.
4. Identify something you love to do. Find a way to fit it into your life.
5. Keep your life simple. Try to be less materialistic and enjoy the more basic things in life, such as by taking long walks in parks and on nature trails.
6. When you have an opportunity to take a nap in the afternoon, go for it. It's a great way to refresh your brain.
7. What you think and how you think affects your general well-being. Try to stay away from negative or self-derogatory thoughts and emotions. This will require practice, but that's okay. In time you will master a new skill and feel better about yourself.
8. Cultivate your spiritual side by keeping in touch with your intuition and your inner self.
9. Eat well and healthy. Buy a new cookbook and try new recipes. Make meals interesting and fun.
10. Plan to exercise regularly. Go for short walks or runs whenever you can. Exercise your eyes regularly, especially if you spend a lot of time in front of the computer. Walk up stairways instead of taking the elevator.
11. Go for regular medical checkups. If you have health problems, talk to your doctor and discuss all of the options available to you.

12. If you have the space, cultivate a garden for vegetables. If you don't have the space, get creative and make some. You can have your garden in small tubs or containers. Also, create an herb garden. Gardening encourages you to be active. It will be relaxing and rewarding to you as you see your plants grow and produce flowers, fruits, and herbs.

13. Take an interest in other people and volunteer in your community.

14. Read books or listen to audio books/CDs/DVDs on self-improvement or on a subject that interests you. Try to learn one new thing every day.

15. Watch comedy movies and shows. A good laugh is great for your mind and your body.

16. Start to pay attention to this moment — your *now*. Whatever you are doing at this time, *do it well*. Whatever you are thinking, *keep an open mind and be curious*.

Congratulations … you are on your way to a FIT Lifestyle!

PART 1

Mental Fitness: Change Your Mind

Power Source Tool #1

Explore Your Mind,
Move Your Body

"The starting point for all achievement is desire. Keep this constantly in mind. Weak desire brings weak results, just as a small amount of fire makes a small amount of heat."

–NAPOLEON HILL

Fitness — mental, physical, and emotional — begins with the mind. It starts with your outlook and motivation.

What does it take to get motivated and make a commitment to fitness?

Ask yourself these questions: How can I change the words I quietly say to myself so I feel more positive about the process? How can I access that inner voice that longs to feel energized mentally, physically, and emotionally?

What's stopping you from getting up each morning excited about the day and looking forward to your workout? What's blocking you from finding that deeply satisfying relationship with fitness?

We all have a desire to be the best we can be, physically and mentally; to feel vital and alive; and to be activated. If you can zone into that power source within you that wants to get fit, then the motivation to achieve that inner desire will just happen. Or will it?

Is there something you would like to try but you just don't know how to get started?

Do you feel a new challenge would be too high a mountain to climb by yourself?

Do you feel you're too old to get going on your fitness goal?

Well, you're not. Finding a connection with fitness and becoming passionate about it is like finding and developing a good relationship. You must be compatible with the fitness environment you choose to spend time in. You must enjoy the activities you participate in. You should experience certain essential qualities in your special connection with fitness, including:

- balance
- confidence
- a level of flexibility
- a willingness to make changes
- a sense of independence and personal growth
- enjoyment — you need to be having some fun.

A passion for fitness doesn't just happen overnight. It may first take the form of morning walks with a friend or perhaps taking the stairs instead of the elevator. Slowly, over time, you will begin to feel energized and motivated to build a stronger relationship with fitness. As you begin to spend more time participating in your new activities, passion will emerge and the desire to make it part of your life will come naturally to you.

Susan's Story

When I joined the YMCA in 2002, I signed up for aerobic fitness classes. From the start I loved the camaraderie of step classes, weights classes, and low-impact classes. In addition, my husband Peter and I attended the Saturday morning Run Fit class together. Although I was always at the back of the running group, walking and jogging while everyone else raced along, I realized how much I enjoyed moving to the music.

After two years of "showing up" at the YMCA, I discovered that jogging, walking, and weights had become my passion. From 2004 to 2007 I progressed from the Saturday Run Fit class to short jogs and long walks. Then I started to compete in races, completing 5k races, 10k races, and half-marathons. In 2004 I won my first medal in a 5k race in Toronto, placing first in my age group. Between 2004 and 2010, I participated in 25 events, ranging from 5k to 42k.

Theresa's Story

Running is the sport I love. It's like having a great relationship. I look forward to reconnecting with it on a regular basis. It rejuvenates me and makes me happier. I feel committed. Running gives me the opportunity to push through my limiting beliefs. It empowers and motivates me. It has expanded my social network.

Reflecting back on my first marathon, I realize I did not have the mindset of a marathoner. The thought of completing 26 miles was far beyond what I believed I was capable of achieving.

To make this breakthrough, I relied on the support of my fellow running friends from a newly formed group I joined back in 1992 called the BTS Road Runners. Doug and Mohamad, and later Dennis, were my running partners. They inspired, encouraged, and trained with me as I prepared for my first two marathons: the Toronto Marathon in September 1992 and the New York City Marathon in October 1992.

THE BENEFITS OF PHYSICAL ACTIVITY AND REGULAR EXERCISE

Although they seem similar in a number of ways, there are differences between physical activity and exercise.

- Physical activity refers to activities that get your body moving, such as gardening, walking the dog, and taking the stairs instead of the elevator.
- Exercise is a form of physical activity that is planned, structured, and repetitive. Examples are weight training, tai chi, and aerobics classes.

Include both in your life. Both will help you to feel better and enjoy life more as you age. Physical activity and exercise together:

- help to prevent or delay many diseases and disabilities
- provide an effective treatment for many chronic conditions
- improve balance and prevent falls
- manage depression, stress, and anxiety and improve your mood
- burn calories, build muscle, reduce fat, and assist with weight management
- increase your energy level
- strengthen your heart, making it more efficient
- lower your blood pressure
- boost HDL (good) cholesterol and aid the circulatory system
- increase flexibility and create stronger bones
- promote better sleep.

LOOK WITHIN TO DISCOVER YOUR FITNESS PASSION

If you are looking for motivation to start (or return to) fitness, ask yourself the following three questions:

1. WHAT DO I WANT TO ACHIEVE THROUGH FITNESS?

Do you believe you can attain your fitness goals? Can you picture where you want to be? Have you taken the time to plan the path to get there? You may not be able to control the outcome of all of life's challenges, but you can choose how you evaluate and grow with each experience.

2. WHY DO I WANT TO ACHIEVE MY FITNESS GOALS?

WHY is it important for you to achieve the goals you have just defined?

Take a few minutes and begin to shape your WHY. Doing this will fuel your desire, determination, and dedication as you pursue your goals. You set goals for a reason, so you need to be clear on why you want to achieve each one. You need to come up with enough compelling reasons to make achieving each goal a priority.

Some reasons may be internal, such as to push yourself, to add to your "bucket list," to accomplish something in your life, to set challenges for yourself, to improve your self-esteem, to develop better coping skills, to manage stress, or to enjoy doing fitness-related activities with family and friends.

Other reasons may be external, such as to lose weight or to impress other people.

You may need both internal and external reasons in order to get, and stay, motivated. Your WHY is what will create your solid foundation.

If your goal is to become motivated to start exercising five days a week, your WHY may be to fit into your old red party dress for the 50th birthday party your husband is throwing for you in three months. Looking great in a dress you haven't put on in years is a strong motivator because with only three months to achieve your goal, you have to get serious about sticking to a new fitness program.

Remember, it has to be a strong WHY, one that will propel you and keep you grounded when you feel like giving up. You just need to have the right combination of reasons to move you in the right direction and stay the course.

Once you have established your WHY, you will encounter three emotional stages as you travel through your fitness journey:

- The first is excitement — you desire the outcome.
- The second is frustration — you think it is too tough.
- The third is satisfaction — experiencing a breakthrough in which you see results and your body starts to respond in positive ways.

3. WHAT CAN HELP ME TO BE INTERNALLY MOTIVATED TO REACH SUCCESS?

Congratulations for defining your WHY. The next step is to understand your Three Internal Drives. These are critical factors for success.

1. Desire

Throughout our journey together in this book, you will complete a number of self-assessment questionnaires and quizzes. You will begin to understand what it's going to take to get *you* moving and find ways to access that power source within *you* that is waiting to come alive. We hope the spark of desire that made you pick up this book and begin to read it ignites into a powerful internal flame of motivation to get fit.

2. Determination

Once you embrace your desire, it is determination and dedication that will carry you to your goal. Keep your mind on what you want to achieve. The relentless quest, the energy that keeps you going day after day, is what will be your determination. If you can stay focused and determined in your quest for your goal, you will succeed.

3. Dedication

Dedication is the price you must pay to achieve what you want. You want to feel good about your body, you want to have energy, and you want to be physically fit. All of this is possible, but you must dedicate a certain amount of time to get what you want. It is easy to dream and it feels good to think of the possibilities. Real change, however, requires a stick-to-it attitude.

You need dedication to move toward your goals. Keep your resolve strong no matter what obstacles get in your way. You can achieve your goal, but you must believe you will succeed.

On a scale from 1 to 10, how dedicated are you, at this moment, to achieving your goal? If your number is not an absolute 10, then you need to go back and revisit your WHY.

SEVEN STRATEGIES FOR DEFINING YOUR FITNESS PASSION

#1. Connect with your talents, strengths, and interests

- How can you apply your existing talents and gifts to a fitness program? Start by viewing fitness activities as acts of expression and originality. For example, gardening is a talent and a creative outlet, as well as an excellent fitness activity. Plant a vegetable garden and an herbs garden and enjoy the rewards of eating fresh produce.

#2. Brainstorm

- Take time to reflect on yourself and your attributes. Get to know yourself. Write down your thoughts and ideas. Look around your house, on your computer, and in your bookshelf for inspiration. Consider activities that fit your health, budget, and lifestyle. You can evaluate them later.
- Novelty can also boost your interest in fitness. Try something unique, such as yoga, spinning, belly dancing, tai chi, synchronized swimming, Frisbee golf, snowshoeing, or kettlebells.

#3. Think about sports and activities you loved doing at other stages in your life

- Did you enjoy bike riding, canoeing, fishing, skating, skiing, or running when you were younger? Did you enjoy jumping rope or playing tennis? Did you like team sports such as baseball, volleyball, or basketball? Think about whether you enjoyed individual activities, two-person activities, or team or group activities. Tap back into that excitement and enthusiasm.
- You're more likely to keep up with a fitness program

that you enjoy. If you love riding your bicycle, consider a spinning class. If you enjoy dancing, an aerobics class that includes dance moves would be a good bet — or a line dancing or Samba class.

#4. Search the Internet for ideas
- Many health, fitness, and consumer websites provide excellent suggestions and ideas related to women, fitness, and health.

#5. Find joy in fitness
- Statements like "I can do this" and "keep going" can become mantras that will help you to pull through the lows and reach new highs.
- Optimism and motivation go hand-in-hand. Visualizing a better you and then actually believing you can get there will give you an internal power source that will help you weather the inevitable motivation droughts that lie ahead.
- Join a laughter yoga group. Since laughter is contagious, it spreads the joy of fitness.

#6. Take the next step
- Assess the strategies and tools in this book and decide what is realistic and available to you.
- Focus on each step of your fitness program, not on how far you have to go to reach your goal. This kind of focus will increase your likelihood of success.
- Share your fitness passion with others who are likely to support you, as well as those who need your help.

#7. Build YOUR perfect FIT relationship
- Think of finding your fitness as being similar to find-

ing your perfect relationship. What do you look for in a good relationship?

1. Compatibility
2. Enjoyment
3. Dedication
4. Connectedness

And when you find that special relationship, you feel activated and full of energy. You can't wait for your next encounter. Well, wouldn't it be great if you could find that kind of FIT in your relationship with fitness? We all tend to have our own unique arousal zone that influences the type of activities we like to do. So if you look at your exercise as a special relationship that is unique to you and that must meet your personal desires and needs, you will see that not every class or routine is going to do it for you. We're here to guide you on the path to finding that special FIT relationship.

OUR POWER SOURCE EXPERT, RUTH KRONGOLD, SPEAKS

Growing up I lacked physical confidence. I developed the kind of shoulder-hunching, nail-picking gawkiness typical of many kids who grow quickly but really have no idea where their arms end or what their body will do next.

I was told I was uncoordinated. Sadly, I spent much of my childhood living down to that label. It is hard to choose from the long list of fitness failures of my youth: the hanging bars I fell off, physical education tests I failed, track and field events I cried through, skates that pinched and impeded glide, a bike that was somehow unstoppable when approaching a field of bricks as I went downhill, bullies I could not outrun who kicked me and taunted me with ethnic slurs, and, alas, a swimming test that I also failed.

Fortunately I had the incredible privilege of spending my summers as a child on the Lake of Bays. There I forged a loving relationship with the clean, clear lake water. I was gratified to find I could stay afloat and paddle my body around for long periods of time. The lake became a place where I was able to be physically active outside the dominant cultural constraints associated with fitness and athleticism.

It seemed miraculous to me that when I was enveloped in the water's embrace I could be as strong, clever, graceful, beautiful, and happy as my imagination allowed. All I had to do was keep going. No competition found its way into this activity, and that suited me just fine. By chance, I discovered the joy fitness can bring through swimming.

As a child with stick-like legs I realized that being able to outrun bullies would have been a useful skill. It was only as a young adult that I realized running toward something is as important as trying to escape. Fitness became associated with pleasure, endurance, and peace. It gives me access to the natural world in ways I am still discovering more than 50 years later, not just as a swimmer, but also as a participant in kayaking, canoeing, snowshoeing, cross-country skiing, and hiking.

Daily distance swimming provides me with foundational strength and endurance. It is a practice that welcomed me back after the births of my two children, bouts of serious illness, surgeries (five in the period of 2002–2003), accidents, divorce, and traumas.

During times of physical and emotional hardship, the memory of feeling free and alive in the water propels me toward continuing the work of rehabilitation.

Pilates and stability ball exercises, along with a grudging minimum of weight training, have given me the strength and flexibility to recover repeatedly from the difficulties life has tossed my way. This hard-won strength gives me the opportunity to support loved ones as they struggle with health issues. I know in my heart I would not be as effective in helping them without the stamina I have gained from consistent efforts to be as mentally and physically fit as I can be.

When I was a student at the University of Toronto, I lived in a dirty rooming house and preferred showering at the local Y, which not only was cleaner but by some small miracle had a pool. Why not swim as well when I was there to shower?

And so I did ... every day. That is how my daily swimming habit began. Whether jumping out of a canoe on a hot summer day and free-styling my way home, doing an early morning triangle swim of our bay accompanied by my family singing to me from a rowboat, or swimming along the shores of wonderful bodies of water, I have always greatly enjoyed connecting with nature through exercise.

OUR POWER SOURCE WOMEN SPEAK

We asked our Power Source Women how they discovered their fitness passion.

Audrey

In the late 1980s, step classes appeared on the scene and I was hooked. Through step I discovered group fitness in its infinite variety and went on to do classes in aerobics, boot camp, circuit training, high intensity interval training, kickboxing, boxing, body sculpting, Pilates, yoga, spinning, and many other disciplines. These days I usually work out five or six days a week for at least a one-hour class, and sometimes twice a day, using a variety of activities.

My love of the moment is boxing, but that could change next week. When it comes to fitness, you have to find what you love and keep doing it until you don't love it any more. Then you can find something else you love to do. In fitness, as in life, there's more than one way to achieve the results you want.

Edna

The turning point for me was six months after my 50th birthday. My son called me from McGill University. He told me he had joined a gym — and I should do the same.

"After all, Mom," he said, "you're middle-aged — you should start to do some exercising."

For some strange reason I took his advice, and joined my local Y. I discovered my fitness passion within one month of joining. After five days of speed walking around the track, I realized I did not enjoy working out alone, so I joined a class — and from that point I became a fitness groupie. I continue to this day to work out in a group setting. There's no doubt about it: The power of the group motivates me.

Since embarking on a regular fitness regime, my body has responded by assuming a more toned appearance. My energy level has increased exponentially.

Psychologically I have acquired a much greater sense of self-esteem and confidence.

Pat

In 1976 I joined CIL Industries and was quickly immersed in a mixed team in the CIL curling culture. The company sponsored instructional sessions and made me a curler, a winter sport I still enjoy today. When I retired from my career 12 years ago, I joined a daytime curling team for women. Curling combines physical activity with socializing. Over the past 10 years I have curled at least twice a week on women's teams and competed in many out-of-club bonspiels.

CIL was a major financial supporter of the North York YMCA in 1979–1980. I joined the Y in 1980 as a charter member and always went there before work. The informal, very early morning group has evolved into many friendships and support groups.

When we were visiting friends in London, Ontario, in 1980, I found out our hostess had organized a fundraising run for their YMCA Shape Up London campaign. I borrowed shorts and shoes from her son and finished the 5k run red and exhausted — and hooked on running.

Phyllis

I was always very fit. I taught Dancercise classes in my early years, until I had a bad fall when I was in my 40s. After the fall, I was disabled for approximately two years and could not walk properly. I had knee surgery when I was 48 and later was diagnosed with scoliosis, fibromyalgia, and a mild case of stenosis.

The day I joined the YMCA in 2004 was the turning point for me. I was 57 years old and wanted so badly to return to exercise. Slowly, my body began to respond positively to the exercise and I reflected back on those days many years earlier when I taught Dancercise.

I wanted to do that again but thought maybe it was too late for me to start given my age. Fortunately, people at the Y supported my idea, and Beth, the staff fitness leader at the Y, gave me a chance to show her what I could do.

I now have my own dance class with a wonderful group of participants. It was the belief other people had in my ability, and, of course, my burning desire to dance that encouraged me to teach a class once a week. I love my newfound fitness.

OUR ROLE MODEL #1: CLAIRE VANDRAMINI

Have you ever had an experience so life changing it transformed the way you did just about everything ever since? Did the same experience help you to develop a passion so great you still work passionately on it every day? Well, that's what happened to me.

MY STORY

I am single, a grandmother, and a homeowner in my 60s. In late May 2009 I was packaged out of a 20-year job. Some changes may be good and some may be very challenging. It's not how or why we get there but how we handle each change that really matters.

Many of us may have to deal with restructuring our days, weeks, or years in a new or different way after a death or divorce; staying excited about our small achievements; or getting over the mourning that comes with a lost future or the loss of a substantial income.

MY WAKE-UP CALL

It happened to me one day when I was on a golf course. When a bunch of cyclists flew by me, all I could think of was, "Why am I here?"

You see, during my husband's illness and leading up to his death in 1999, I had started to cycle just to get away from all the stress and hurt we both felt throughout his cancer treatments.

After my husband's decline into death, an 18-month period of living hell, I purchased a road bike with the full knowledge I might not be able to keep up with anyone who could ride with one leg.

MY SOLUTION

I went on a trip to Italy with some of the finest amateur cyclists I've ever known. One of the women, Louise McGonigal, won the Ironman Hawaii in her age category (65+) and set a world record in the Lake Placid Ironman in 2008. This trip to Italy was my very first alone. Was I scared? You bet. This trip taught me independence — that I could leap into the unknown and not be too afraid. I was 51.

Several years later, I joined the YMCA in Toronto and started running with the Tuesday and Thursday Northern Backwards bunch. Was I scared? You bet. Could I keep up? No. Did I get dropped from the pack? Yes. Running is really tough, but running at the Y with a team makes all the difference. When you show you're committed to the group and want to be part of it, you become one of them. All you need is a good pair of running shoes and a willingness to do your best to keep up with them at 6:10 in the morning.

Knowing these people and joining their running culture helped me find the courage to enter my first road races. Their support of my efforts to participate in triathlons is one of the reasons I'm working so hard. This group taught me the importance of being part of a team. The race strategy the team provided me with helped me win second place in my first 10k race in 2008. I was 60.

MY FITNESS ROUTINE

This brings me to the last leg of my decision to try competing in triathlons. Before I started swimming on a regular basis three years ago at the Y, I thought jumping off and paddling back to a dock was swimming. Now, I'm training to do 2k in the water in less than 40 minutes. The discipline of swimming has taught me to never give up. To never get down on myself and to know that quality is far superior to quantity.

THE RESULT

So, what have I done thus far? I've been to Italy twice, Portugal once, Mallorca, Spain, twice, and Florida twice — each time with my bike, my running shoes, and my wetsuit. I've competed in three cycling races, four road races, and many short triathlons. In July 2009 I completed my first Half Ironman in Peterborough and finished second in my age category. In September 2009 I traveled to the Gold Coast of Australia for the World Triathlon Championships – Olympic Division. My goal in 2011 is to complete my first full Ironman and get my "finisher" Ironman tattoo.

WHAT I LEARNED

Each of us can excel in anything we try if we're willing to explore what it is we are truly passionate about.

Everyone can develop a fitness passion.

ANSWER CLAIRE VANDRAMINI'S FITNESS PASSION QUESTIONS

1. When you were young, did you ever participate in a sport you really enjoyed or excelled at?

2. Can you describe a physical activity you really enjoyed doing yesterday or even last week?

3. Do you think you could turn your interest in a specific sport activity (e.g., swimming, yoga, etc.) into a lifestyle change that could help improve your overall health and well-being?

4. Do your friends ever mention how happy you are when you talk about your involvement with a specific exercise or sport?

5. What plan can you make so you can devote a part of each day or week to a real fitness endeavor?

Make a Fitness Pact with yourself. The world and your family need people who have come alive by being more active. What's holding you back?

We're pleased to pass you on for the remainder of this chapter to journaling expert Lesley Shore, whose words of wisdom and gentle journaling advice appear at the end of each chapter. We suggest you start a notebook for journaling.

JOURNALING WITH LESLEY SHORE

"A journey of a thousand miles begins with a single step." –Lao-tzu

Once when I was seven I was riding my bike on the sidewalk of the quiet Winnipeg street where I grew up, and Claudia, the tough girl at the end of the block, put her hand on my bike's rear tire. I catapulted over the front of my bike. As a result of my fall I got a blood clot in my foot. I sat propped up on pillows with my leg elevated for a week to prevent the clot from traveling to my heart or lungs.

I was an only child who arrived late in my parents' marriage. They treated me like a china doll. "Be careful" was the constant refrain of my mother, father, and doting grandma, who lived with us. That accident with the bike sealed the deal on my athletic career. I wasn't to have one.

Though I was tall, I was the last one to be chosen for teams. It didn't take long for me to determine I didn't have much to contribute. In grade 5, while the other kids played baseball, Mary Van Buskirk and I lolled about in left field searching for daisies to weave into chains.

My mother had been athletic in her youth. She had two athletic brothers. But I was groomed to be a good student. Books were my constant companions. I was quiet like my dad, who couldn't get into the army because he had poor vision and flat feet, just like me.

Well into her 70s my mother was an avid walker. I knew she walked to work out the disappointments of her life. Friends would say, "I saw your mother walking last week. Boy, she goes at quite a clip." It was not unusual for her to walk for miles all the way downtown to do her volunteer work and then halfway back again. She never grew old. At 80 she got cancer and days after her 81st birthday she was gone.

Walking was her legacy to me. You don't have to be the least bit athletic to walk. You don't have to belong to a gym. For 30 years, off and on, I've been walking the neighborhood ravine. It's 45 minutes, round-trip. I can do it summer and winter, weather permitting.

I wish I could tell you I'm disciplined enough to do the walk every day of the week. Because now, at 63, I have the time to do so. But I don't.

That's my goal as I write the journal sections of this book: to stick to my own exercise routine of regular walking. I plan to add some weights and stretches, maybe even a bit of running. My older daughter is getting married in six months. My plan is to have Michelle Obama's arms by then.

Commitment to a fitness routine begins in the mind. But exercise enhances all parts of our selves. The women you meet in this book have one thing in common: discipline. Many are at the gym at six a.m. because they want to do it.

I could never do that. Maybe you couldn't either. Discipline for me means holding myself responsible to exercise five or more times a week, sometimes for 45 minutes each time, sometimes for only 20.

I'm a lone exerciser who has always felt awkward in classes. I was 21 before I mastered which was my right and which was my left hand. In university, where a gym class was compulsory, I chose golf. Classes were held in a gym where we gathered on the perimeter of the gleaming wood floor and aimed our clubs up into the pyramided stands.

I decided if I followed the teacher around as she advised girl after girl on her swing, she would never actually get to watch me. I can't imagine how that teacher chose a grade for me. She'd never seen me swing. But I was the one who lost out. I wish I had started to learn to golf then.

Some mornings it takes a lot of effort for me to literally throw myself out the door for my walk. But within 60 seconds I begin to enjoy myself. I love filling my lungs with the fresh air of the neighborhood ravine after so many years of sitting in front of a computer in stale offices or breathing the heavy air of overpopulated classrooms.

START JOURNALING

Set a timer and write for 20 minutes in your FIT Journal about your own past history with exercise and fitness. Allow your mind to roam free and jot down the memories that float up.

Remember, what you write in this journal is for your eyes alone. No teacher will be grading you. What do you bring to this journey? What drew you to this book? The past is always present. How is that so for you?

Power Source Tool #2

Do Your Research

"Take the first step in faith. You don't have to
see the whole staircase, just the first step."

–DR. MARTIN LUTHER KING JR.

Part of developing a positive attitude toward fitness is doing your own research. What is your current fitness level? What are your fitness needs? What types of exercise programs are recommended for women in your situation and with your needs and aspirations?

As you do your research, your knowledge, comfort level, and experience will expand. You will develop a more natural connection to your own fitness. Doing research will help you make informed choices as you plan your new lifestyle. It will be a rewarding process: As you build the foundation of your knowledge, your goals will take shape.

Read magazines and books, tap into the Internet, connect with people, and stay committed to your personal growth and a fitter, healthier you. Continue to do research as you improve your physical health and lifestyle. This will help your mind open up to the fitness options that are right for you.

Susan's Story

In 2005 I heard about a trainer, Chen Cohen, who was preparing 10 men for the Chicago Marathon. I was intrigued by the idea of completing a marathon and wanted to ask him to train me as well. However, I knew nothing about marathons and decided to do some research before talking to him.

First, I made a list of potential marathons by location, by degree of difficulty, by cost, by season, by beauty of location, and by criteria to enter. I read books and magazines related to marathons and women's fitness. I also attended consumer shows related to sports, women, fitness, and running.

Next, I visited running stores and talked to staff and customers. I looked at their equipment, clothing, books, and clinics. I joined a free walking group once a week for companionship and motivation.

I talked to people who had completed marathons and asked them about their problems and successes.

Finally, I looked on the Internet for marathon websites and blogs, as well as articles, tips, and free newsletters related to jogging, walking, and running.

Theresa's Story

I took an interest in health at an early age when I realized I was the one who was ultimately responsible for the well-being of my own mind and body. Two books I read when I was 18 changed the direction of my relationship with food. They were *Fit for Life*, by Harvey and Marilyn Diamond, and *Diet for a New America*, by John Robbins.

Today I continue my journey to educate myself on mind-and-body health issues. My understanding of how stress affects my body allows me to fine-tune my nutritional plan whenever my physical and/or mental demands increase. The knowledge and experience I have gained over the years give me the tools I need to make positive changes in my life and enable me to be a source of guidance for others.

SEVEN STRATEGIES FOR RESEARCHING FITNESS

#1. Visit bookstores, video stores, and libraries
Buy (or borrow from the library) the best fitness-related books and magazines available in order to find tips, suggestions, race schedules, and training advice. Trade exercise videos or DVDs with a friend so you don't get bored.

#2. Search the Internet for fitness templates, downloads, apps, and videos
Websites are convenient ways to expand your knowledge base, get free advice, and find a community of people committed to fitness.
- Surf food-related websites to get recipes for healthy meals and snacks.
- Sign up for free newsletters or blogs related to fitness.
- Enroll in an online coaching program.
- Look at online fitness video games:
  - Investigate Nintendo's Wii video games, including bowling, tennis, boxing, and baseball.
  - Also look at Wii Fit for more activities, including yoga, aerobics, and strength training, which are all done on a board that connects to your Nintendo Wii console. You can even check your body mass index and weight and track your progress as you advance in the game. Nintendo DS allows you to hook up a pedometer to the system and access diet tips and health trivia.

- Interactive games like Dance Dance Revolution, Wii Sports, and even Rock Band can improve your health and motor skills.
- Fitbit (www.fitbit.com) allows you to keep on top of your fitness regimen online. In addition, a community function allows you to connect with your family and friends if you want to get in shape together — at least virtually.
- The Expresso Fitness Virtual Reality Bike brings excitement to the sometimes monotonous experience of stationary biking by using TV screens that add a video game to your pedaling. In addition, workout information can be uploaded to the Internet and you can track your progress.

#3. Visit fitness-related retail outlets and online fitness outlets
Sign up for free sports clinics. You can join a training program for an event and look at their workout clothes, equipment, books, and magazines. Talk to the staff. Don't be afraid to ask questions.

Clean out your closet and donate any clothes, including fitness gear, that you have not worn in the past year. ✪

Buy recycled workout clothes for biking, running, hiking, climbing, paddling, and yoga from stores or online. Look for clothes made with organic cotton, hemp, bamboo, and recycled or soy fibers. These fibers are usually grown and harvested in a sustainable manner. ✪

Look for barely used fitness items such as exercise DVDs, home gym equipment, and similar items at yard sales or garage sales, or on Internet community boards. ✪

Trade in old, worn-out sneakers for fitness shoes related to your exercise program. Or find a pair of gently used shoes. ✦

#4. Look at fitness facilities, golf courses, community centers, and women-only fitness centers

Search for the best programs and instructors related to your fitness passion. The right teacher can give you the best level of understanding necessary to enjoy an activity.

For indoor activities, look into water aerobics classes. Water aerobics is an activity you can enjoy for life.

Also, investigate outdoor activity areas in your community such as nature trails, parks, climbing walls, and hiking paths.

#5. Explore ways to set up a space for a home gym in your house, condo, or apartment

If you're planning to invest in exercise equipment, choose pieces that are practical, enjoyable, and easy to use. Try the equipment out at a fitness center before buying your own. In the chapter *Power Source Tool #7*, we suggest some equipment you can buy or make for your home gym.

If your budget allows it, hire a trainer to set up your home program for you, recommend the equipment appropriate to achieving your goals, and correct your form.

#6. Attend consumer shows related to health, lifestyle, fitness, and/or women

Look at the products they display and sell, talk to the exhibitors, and take their literature home to study.

#7. Register for special events, such as races, competitions, and tournaments

A scheduled event will keep you motivated and committed, and you will have the benefit of learning something new as you train.

Research a 5k walk or run, a swim competition, a golf tournament, or a bicycle competition to raise money, challenge yourself, and have fun.

Form a team for a charity event with a partner, family, friends, or colleagues. It's a great way to meet your own fitness goals while enjoying time with others.

SEVEN STRATEGIES FOR DEVELOPING NUTRITIONAL FITNESS

An enormous amount of information is available on nutrition and diet. It can all seem overwhelming and at times even conflicting. How can you eat for optimal health or weight loss? Begin by striving for balance in your diet. Decide what you need to do to achieve a healthy lifestyle. Below are some tips that will help you to kick-start your healthy-eating lifestyle.

#1. Read the labels

Educate yourself about what's in your food by reading the labels. Don't be fooled by thinking you can eat more of a low-fat food: chances are it contains just as many calories. Look at things like fiber, protein, and sugar content to help guide your decisions.

#2. Drink more water

Your body needs water to function. Many parts of your body contain water, including blood, lean muscle, and even your brain.

Water in your body serves to:
- regulate body temperature
- carry nutrients from food and oxygen to the cells
- remove wastes from the body
- cushion joints.

Tips to get you to drink more water:
- Keep it handy. If you carry water with you, you will be more likely to drink it. If you work in an office, keep a bottle of water on your desk so it's within reach. At home, keep it near your computer and television, and throughout your house. Have a bottle by your side in the car. Put water in as many places as you can so it always catches your eye.
- Ask for water when you go out for a meal. Request it with a slice of lemon or lime.
- Stop buying water in plastic bottles and invest in an eco-friendly water bottle. You can purchase a water bottle online or at your favorite health food store. So many interesting colors and designs are available. Find one that is visually exciting and go from a dull, environmentally unfriendly plastic water bottle to a cool, environmentally friendly drinking experience. ✤
- Make your water more interesting. If you don't like the taste of water on its own, try adding a light splash of lemon or lime juice. Another great way to make drinking water fun is to freeze bits of peeled lemons,

limes, oranges, or even strawberries and use them as ice cubes. Adding a little mint to your water can also be very refreshing. Have fun with your water and you will begin to enjoy drinking it.

#3. Eat at least one serving of fruits or vegetables with each meal and snack

Fruits and vegetables should make up a large portion of your diet. These colorful and sometimes crunchy foods are low in calories and high in vitamins, minerals, phytochemicals, and fiber. Experts suggest eating five to nine servings of fruits and vegetables every day.

- Buy fresh, local, and organic foods from farmers' markets and co-ops whenever possible. Ⓖ
- Start your own vegetable garden and enjoy the results. Ⓖ
- Grow your own herbs in a small herb garden in your kitchen window. Use them to season your foods. Ⓖ

Tips to help you reach your quota of fruits and vegetables each day:

- Fill a bowl with different fruits such as apples and oranges and place it on the counter for easy access. Eat fruits and vegetables that are in season whenever possible.
- Cut up veggies and fruits for quick snacks, putting them in handy resealable plastic bags.
- When you are steaming veggies, cook extra portions for snacks.
- Eat more salads. They are quick and easy to make. Add variety to your salads by spicing them up with a

mixture of dried or fresh fruits and vegetables, either cooked or raw. Add a little goat's cheese and olive oil to the mix for interest.

- Try out new fruits or vegetables, such as jicama, plantain, starfruit, or bok choy. ⊛
- Instead of eating out, bring a healthy, low-calorie lunch to work. ⊛

#4. Eat more whole-grain foods

All types of grains are good sources of complex carbohydrates and various vitamins and minerals. Grains that are not refined, or whole grains, are a good source of important nutrients, such as selenium, potassium, and magnesium. They are also a great source of fiber to help you keep your digestive tract healthy.

Examples of whole grains include barley, brown rice, buckwheat, oatmeal, popcorn, wild rice, and whole-wheat bread or pasta.

Tips to help you get enough of your daily grains:

- *Breakfast*: For a quick and easy breakfast, pour milk, soya milk, or almond milk over a bowl of ready-to-eat whole-grain cereal (an unsweetened, low-fat variety). To ensure that the cereal is packed full of nutrients, choose one with at least three to five grams of fiber per serving.
- *Lunch*: Pick up a pack of whole-grain or whole-wheat pita bread and create a quick, delicious, and nutritious wrap by whipping up a salad full of vegetables with perhaps an added can of tuna fish. Toss it on the bread, wrap it up, and enjoy.
- *Snacks*: Try whole-rye crackers with a spoonful of fruit jam or hummus. You will be getting a power-

house snack that will be satisfying and nutritious while keeping your blood sugar stable until mealtime. Did you know that popcorn is a whole grain and a great snack? Just make sure to use kernels that you pop yourself in a pan, not the ready-to-eat popcorn in a package. A cup of popcorn can be a nice treat, especially when you sprinkle a little sea salt, a little garlic powder, or your favorite spice on top.

- *Dinner*: Make sure you buy whole-wheat pastas and not refined white noodles. Cook up a pot of whole-wheat pasta; add vegetables and tomato sauce and let it simmer. This is a great way for you to get your veggies and whole grains in one recipe.

#5. Eat lean meats and alternatives

Proteins are the building blocks for just about everything in your body from enzymes and hormones to bones, muscles, and skin.

The recommended daily allowance of protein for women is approximately 10–35% of total daily calories. Based on this RDA, women beginning at age 19 require approximately 46 grams of protein. But factors such as level of activity and current health condition could influence your needs.

Foods that contain protein include eggs, cheese, many types of legumes, and meat. Be sure to avoid meats that are fatty. Replace them with lean meats such as chicken, flank steak, lean ground beef, or fish.

Buy fresh and lean red meat and poultry from a local butcher (organic, if possible).

#6. Choose low-fat dairy products
The suggested daily intake of low-fat dairy products is indicated as three servings a day for the average adult.

Low-fat dairy products have less saturated fat.

Many studies have shown the health benefits of low-fat dairy products. They are beneficial when you are trying to lose weight because of their reduced caloric content. Low-fat dairy products help lower blood pressure and, in turn, help reduce the risk of heart ailments.

Studies have also shown that low-fat dairy products help to lower LDL cholesterol levels, reduce risk of hypertension, and promote healthy thyroid functioning. Low-fat, skim, or one-percent milk, low-fat cottage cheese, and low-fat yogurt are a few examples of low-fat dairy products.

#7. Choose the best fat options and limit your sweets
When choosing fats, your best options are unsaturated fats: monounsaturated and polyunsaturated fats. These fats have the positive effect of helping to lower your risk of heart disease by reducing the levels of cholesterol and low-density lipoprotein (LDL) in your blood.

Here are the best food sources of healthy fats:
- monounsaturated fat: olive oil, canola oil, avocados, nuts, and seeds
- polyunsaturated fat: vegetable oils (such as safflower, corn, sunflower, soy, and cottonseed oils), nuts, and seeds
- Omega-3 fatty acids: fatty cold-water fish (salmon, mackerel, and herring), flaxseed, flax oil, and walnuts.

(Note: A great website that will help you learn more about your daily requirements based on the Recommended Dietary Allowance Guide is www.fnic.nal.usda.gov. [Click on "Dietary Guidance."] You can customize your daily requirements on the site based on your age and level of activity and whether you are looking to maintain, gain, or lose weight. Explore and enjoy this site and get vital information that will add value to your healthy living food plan.)

It's hard to imagine a sugar-free life. Well, you don't need to cut sugar out of your life completely. Here are a few ways to satisfy your sweet tooth.

- Clean out your cupboards. Do not store any high-calorie foods in your home. Get rid of foods that are not on your preferred list and that you will be tempted to eat. It's best to have cupboards full of healthy food in order to avoid temptation. Also, try switching to unsweetened cereals and jams.
- Find alternatives. Sugar is an appetite stimulator: the more you eat, the more you crave. Substitute healthy treats for sweet treats, such as smoothies made with fruit, or frozen fruit bars made from fresh fruit.
- Try fruit for dessert topped with a couple of spoonfuls of yogurt.
- Handle your food cravings. If you start to long for an unhealthy sweet, go for a walk, read a book, take a bath, or make a telephone call. Do something to distract yourself from thinking about the craving.
- Do not skip meals. This helps to keep your blood sugar stable and will save you from craving sweets throughout the day.
- Find a good substitute. Pop a mint in your mouth when you feel the need for something sweet. Mints offer a little sweetness with fewer calories.

Finally, here are two important tips for optimal digestion:

- Chew your food. Chewing is the first step in the diges-
  tive process. When you put food into your mouth and
  begin chewing (also known as masticating), the smaller
  pieces are mixed with a digestive enzyme and the pro-
  cess begins. Digestion is the process of extracting what
  is good from your food and expelling the leftovers. Pay
  attention to the textures and flavors of your food.
- The next time you eat, slow down and think about
  the process. Sit down and breathe properly. Make
  sure you're thoroughly chewing each bite to get the
  maximum nutrition out of each morsel.

A FINAL WORD ON NUTRITIONAL FITNESS AND FOOD

As you continue your research, you'll see that healthy eating is only half of the healthy lifestyle equation. Incorporate your fitness into this plan on a regular basis. Your body requires enough good food daily to nourish your cells and provide you with the amount of fuel energy you need.

You should be low on fuel reserves at the end of the day because your body is preparing to rest. When you sleep, your body goes through a rejuvenation process. This process does not function optimally when food is present. Experts advise against eating a meal before bedtime. If you must eat then, try to stick to fruit. By maximizing your body's sleep rejuvenation time, you will find you awaken more refreshed both mentally and physically.

At this point, as a result of your research, you are increasing your commitment to making lifestyle changes. The basic health tips in this chapter will give you a great start toward improved health. Remember to go at your own pace and make the changes that fit your lifestyle. Enjoy the process and experiment with different foods. Make it fun and interesting.

OUR POWER SOURCE EXPERT,
RUTH KRONGOLD, SPEAKS

Basic knowledge of physiology is very useful in understanding the physical changes that occur unbidden throughout the stages of life — and in developing strategies to maximize fitness results in spite of these changes.

I have expanded my learning opportunities along the way by consulting experienced people in my chosen fitness endeavors, by reading, and by watching videos of the experts.

When I was recovering from injuries and health setbacks, I researched and trained in Pilates and stability ball exercises. This helped me to rebuild my core strength and return to endurance activities.

Today, the encroachment of arthritis, including pain, challenges me to research exercises, diet, and medical treatments that will enable me to continue an active lifestyle.

OUR POWER SOURCE WOMEN SPEAK

We asked our Power Source Women to share the kinds of research they did for their fitness endeavors.

Audrey

I did a little research into sports clubs and found one that was a good fit for me at the time. It has since been sold and I have joined a new club. A benefit of group fitness is you can rely on the instructors' training and knowledge, which is likely to be thorough and up-to-date. Eventually I learned that the main components of fitness were cardio, strength, and flexibility. I try to incorporate all three into the classes I choose.

Edna

I was very lucky — I live close by the gym so I did not have to do any research to find a facility that worked for me.

Pat

I decided I wanted to get back to serious running last year. A trainer, Chen Cohen, leads a women's running club for mature women in midtown Toronto and I joined. Many of the women train for races. Chen has helped me to improve my endurance and avoid injury.

Phyllis

I attended dance fitness classes and evaluated what people liked. I watched and I listened, then I developed my own style of dance class. I believe people like to move their bodies and listen to good music — it's a great recipe for energizing your mind and your body.

JOURNALING WITH LESLEY SHORE

"We are all pilgrims on the same journey …
but some pilgrims have better road maps." –Nelson DeMille

Like Theresa, I read *Fit for Life* many years ago. That, coupled with the later discovery that I had inherited polycystic kidney disease from my father, prompted me to eat nutritiously and drink lots of water. I happen to love fruit, veggies, and grains. Large servings of protein aren't good for me, but they've never appealed to me either. My mother always kept a cupboard brimming with cookies and candy bars that I was free to enjoy in moderation. I was grateful for her attitude and took the same approach with my own children.

I love walking alone but at the suggestion of Susan Sommers I have begun to change my routine a bit. My first purchase was a Wii Fit at Costco. I snapped it up without realizing I needed a Wii console to use it. It was too much of an investment for me at that point in my journey, so instead I invested modestly in exercise equipment and DVDs purchased at Winners, a local discount department store. I work with a weighted ball and use resistance bands and three-pound weights that came with a Pilates DVD. I've become addicted to the weighted ball and even managed to get my 27-year-old daughter, a novice gym rat, to admit it's a quick, effective, fun routine.

Susan and Theresa offer many suggestions in this chapter. Some will appeal to you more than others. I'm thinking of trying a yoga class right in my neighborhood. How about you?

START JOURNALING

Write in your FIT Journal for 20 minutes (using the timer if it helps) about the kind of fitness research you might like to do and how you think this would help you on your journey. How about a salsa class? Bought new running shoes yet?

Don't be afraid to dream big. Nobody's watching but you.

Power Source Tool #3

Build Your Accountability Team

"Every one of us gets through the tough times
because somebody is there, standing in
the gap to close it for us."

–OPRAH WINFREY

In the previous two chapters we looked at the process of changing your mind about fitness and researching fitness as it relates to you. Now that you're beginning to exercise and are watching what you eat, you need to be accountable — to yourself and others.

In fact, personal accountability hinges on having an accountability team: people who believe in you, motivate you, want you to succeed, and check your progress on a regular basis. This chapter shows the importance of such a team to your mental fitness, which of course translates into physical fitness.

As studies show, people who take classes with other people, join a team, connect through e-mail and online coaching, or work out with other people have the highest fitness success rates. Surround yourself with people who exercise regularly. You can keep in touch with your accountability team in person, by phone, through e-mail, on Facebook, or with Twitter.

Seek out people who have the energy you want and get them to describe their motivation. Ask, listen, and observe. Build trust and honesty into these relationships.

You can even create a Fitness Pact to keep you motivated and committed. An excellent example of these pacts is available for downloading from *Experience Life* magazine's website: www.experiencelifemag.com. Feel free to customize it so it works for you and your fellow pact participants.

Susan's Story

Over the years I have always had a strong support system for fitness, including my family, friends, and colleagues.

In my 30s I belonged to a wonderful women-only fitness facility and I developed friendships through the fitness classes I attended. I also loved swimming laps in their heated indoor pool and relaxing in a warm robe.

When I decided to sign up for marathons in 2005 and 2007, I found an inspirational team of people to share my dream with me. The team included two trainers, Beverly Tyler and Chen Cohen. They created fitness programs for me that included weights training, walking, jogging, and stretching. They also went outdoors with me once a week for short runs and hills.

In 2005 one of my closest friends, Pat McMonagle, said she would go out with me once a week to help me to prepare for my marathon. In the end Pat joined me at both marathons and talked me through the last 10k to the finish lines. To this day, Pat and I still go out every Tuesday morning at 5:30 a.m. for a walk or jog. Now both of us compete in half-marathons.

My two daughters joined me and cheered me on as I ran my marathons. Andrea, 39, met me at 20 kilometers and ran for an hour and a half. Danielle, 37, was waiting for me at the finish line. My husband, Peter, met me at 37 kilometers and helped Pat bring me in.

I continue to work out on my own every Saturday morning. I take a one- or two-hour walk or jog, as part of my half-marathon training. I vary my routes, which gives me a chance to relax, meditate, and enjoy the gorgeous scenery.

Theresa's Story

Exercise played a big part in helping me deal with the stresses I faced growing up with parental uncertainty. I joined my first gym when I was an adolescent. I hired my first personal trainer at the age of sixteen. I had a part-time job, attended school, and visited the gym regularly. The gym environment reinforced my committment to a healthy lifestyle and helped me to connect with people with a positive mindset. It was the beginning of a mindset I would grow to love.

As a young woman, I continued my journey to a greater understanding of health by visiting a wide variety of alternative health-care practitioners and sampling many natural remedies.

I started to run marathons in 1992 when I became a member of a new running group called the BTS Road Runners. (I later was honored to become the group's president.)

As I expanded my running community, I had the good fortune to meet another outstanding group of runners called the Rocky Road Runners. Recently I had the honor of participating with them in Issie's Quest. Issie is a man who after battling cancer made a pledge to run 60 marathons by his 60th birthday, raising funds for cancer research. His 60th marathon was at Niagara-on-the-Lake. Issie celebrated his victory that afternoon with all of us. (Go to http://pmhf3.akaraisin.com/common/Event/About.aspx?seid=2592&mid=58.)

This was a running event that went far beyond completing a race and collecting a medal at the end. Issie's Quest created a cohesiveness of spirit in those of us who ran with him that day. His quest and his victory made running a marathon secondary to why we were there.

This is an example of how the power of belonging to a

like-minded fitness community can help you to endure physical feats because of the greater good you are committed to. Community can provide the inspiration and the support we need as we travel on our fitness journey.

I have also had the privilege of running with another amazing group of people called the North York YMCA Northern Backwards runners, but the two men who have continued to be my good running friends when I am not connecting with one of my running groups are Peter and Alfred.

Running with like-minded individuals or groups helps me in powerful ways. This accountability network keeps me committed, inspires me (feeds my motivation), and supports me (giving me encouragement that can break limiting beliefs).

It also socializes me as I develop new friendships with people who have strong interests in common.

SEVEN STRATEGIES FOR BUILDING YOUR ACCOUNTABILITY TEAM

#1. Do something for yourself
Make fitness a top priority in your life. Schedule fitness the way you would arrange an important meeting or appointment. It is a priority on par with work, family, and other commitments. Block off times for physical activity on a regular basis and make sure your friends, family, and colleagues are aware of your commitment. Pay attention to your own needs.

#2. Find people to support you. Offer your support to others
Spend time with the people you want to emulate. Share your fitness goals, passion, and dreams with people who are likely to support you. Encourage them to offer help and inspiration and to ask you about your progress. That kind of support and leverage will keep you motivated.

The social aspect of an accountability team can uplift you and break down any feelings of isolation. Find someone you are comfortable with and make dates for walks or workouts at the gym.

Look around your gym or fitness classes to find people who are struggling. Do you see newcomers who can't figure out how to use the equipment? Offer to help them, or volunteer to teach a yoga class to friends or co-workers.

#3. Make exercise and fitness activities a family affair

Ask your partner, spouse, or children to share your activities. Use the weekends to bike ride, ice skate, play tennis, bowl, golf (or miniature golf), jog, or walk as a family.

#4. Create a walking group

Ask your friends, family members, people from your neighborhood, or colleagues at work to join you. Find people with similar goals, such as losing weight, enjoying nature, starting a jogging routine, or hiking.

Decide when, where, and how often you will walk and whether you will walk outdoors or indoors. Map out your routes and continue to add distance and increase the level of difficulty.

Prepare the right equipment for walking: a pedometer (your goal should be ten thousand steps each day), an appropriate type of shoe, identification, a water bottle, cash, a cell phone, and a map.

After each walk, gather for a healthy breakfast, lunch, or latte at a local restaurant or cafe.

Keep track of your progress in your Weekly FIT Training Log (see the chapter *Power Source Tool #7*), including the distance you walked, how long it took, the difficulty of your route, and your level of enjoyment.

#5. Sign up for a team sport or a league

Join a curling club, a hiking club, a cycling group, or a running group. The expectations of others can push you to succeed. Hard work and self-improvement are great motivators but the drive to keep up with others will encourage you to increase your level of activity.

#6. Join an online community or blog

Look for people with goals, activities, and motivation similar to yours.

#7. Hire a personal trainer, coach, or mentor to get you started and to keep you on track

Hire a certified expert to provide a personalized assessment and to develop a realistic plan to achieve your fitness, health, and/or weight-loss goals.

If possible, get a referral from someone you know who works with the trainer. An experienced trainer can sense the need for minor or major changes in the frequency, intensity, and duration of your fitness program. He or she can provide a stronger foundation by teaching you proper exercise form.

Ask for a résumé and evaluate the person's education in exercise science or medicine, certification from an accredited organization, up-to-date knowledge and skills, experience with people your age, and experience with people with medical conditions. Ask for references.

Here are some things to consider when selecting and working with a personal trainer: What is the personality of the trainer? Does he or she listen to you, explain everything clearly, feel passionate about their work, motivate you, and have a sense of humor?

> To cut costs, share personal training sessions with your partner, friends, or colleagues.

OUR POWER SOURCE EXPERT, RUTH KRONGOLD, SPEAKS

I get a lot of support from my family and friends, in particular, my daughter. She and I have a reciprocal relationship, supporting each other through good times and bad. She is there when the waters get rough, sharing her confidence in me and reminding me that all of our life journeys are undertaken one stroke, one step, and one moment at a time.

Right now I am struggling to use my custom-molded knee brace to hike, cross-country ski, and snowshoe. It is rigid and cumbersome but is essential for my mobility as my knees continue to deteriorate. The thought of losing mobility both terrifies and saddens me, and my daughter encourages me not to give up. She is a trailblazer in the woods around our cottage, increasing my feeling of security and enjoyment as I continue to traverse those paths.

Both my son and daughter have always encouraged me to take that morning walk or go for a swim when I seem a bit grouchy. They know I will feel better when I return.

Coaches and lifeguards have been wonderful supporters as well, offering expertise, help, and friendship when I need it.

Occasionally I am surprised and heartened by strangers who notice the length of time I have been in the water and feel motivated to add a few more lengths to their workout.

OUR POWER SOURCE WOMEN SPEAK

We asked our Power Source Women to tell us about the people on their accountability team and how they keep in touch with them.

Audrey

Accountability in group fitness means showing up for the particular classes or instructors you've agreed to work with. I keep copies of my fitness schedule everywhere and don't miss many of my favorite classes when I'm in town.

It's harder when I travel, which I do quite often. I usually pack my iPod and a skipping rope. One of my instructors was kind enough to load some step music on my iPod. I can do my own step class wherever I can find a step. I really, really hate machines so I avoid them at all costs.

Edna

My support system is made up of my family — my brothers and their wives, my son and daughter-in-law — and my friends, men and women both married and single. I keep in touch with all of these by e-mail or voice-mail. I don't take any of my friends for granted. I see them on a regular basis, some more than others, but we always have a sense of what's going on in each other's lives.

Pat

Curling and running have provided me with lasting friendships. I still get together with people I curled with years ago and enjoy weekends away with my current curling teammates. I also love the ongoing contact with my running buddies and my coach.

Phyllis

Fitness has enhanced my daily level of functioning. I have also made many new friends. Having fitness in my life has kept my mood up and given me the strength to enjoy each day.

I value my YMCA friends, the participants in my dance class, and the leadership staff person, Beth, who believed in me and gave me a chance to demonstrate that I still had what it takes, 30 years later, to teach a dance class again.

OUR ROLE MODEL #2: MAUREEN CATANIA

I was nearly 40 before I developed a weight problem. Until that time I thought I was blessed with the mythological gene enabling you to eat anything without gaining an ounce.

And I do mean anything. It wasn't uncommon for me in my youth to have a chocolate bar and coffee for breakfast, followed by a cigarette or two. Not to mention my love of birthday cake — and it didn't matter if it wasn't my birthday.

For so many years my bad eating behavior continued to reward me. I am five-foot-two and at the time was 95 pounds. I coasted along without a concern about any threats to my size two waistline. Other people needed to watch their weight, count calories, power walk, and generally deny themselves the pleasure of foods. Not me.

MY WAKE-UP CALL

Then, like Humpty Dumpty, my concept of who I was came crashing down around me. I was 46 when the wake-up call came loud and clear. Someone reminded me that both of my parents died in their early 50s and that I shouldn't tempt fate by carrying around so much extra weight.

By my mid-40s I was no longer hovering around the 100-pound mark. I had ballooned to 171 pounds. And I was in serious denial about it. After discovering I had hypothyroidism, I came to the conclusion I was always going to struggle with my weight. The revelation was bittersweet: I now felt I had the perfect excuse for being fat.

I became used to the side effects of being overweight: the shortness of breath, acid reflux after eating, snoring in my sleep, aches and pains everywhere, and mental fogginess. I had a poor self-image. Health-wise I was falling apart.

MY SOLUTION

To regain control of my life, I embarked on a two-tier weight-loss program that included losing weight with the help of Herbal Magic and joining the Fitness Clubs of Canada.

After joining Herbal Magic and reviewing the eating program with the HM coach, I wondered how I could eat so little and not feel starved.

I had to retrain my brain and my stomach to eat healthier than I had been doing, and to control my portions.

Within a few short weeks on the HM program, I discovered where the magic was. By following the prescribed eating plan — which includes a daily balance of protein, starch, fruits, vegetables, dairy, and healthy fats, plus plenty of water along with the natural supplements — I was no longer hungry all the time. I found I could actually stick to the program and not cheat. Each week I lost weight.

What helped me stay the course was the constant monitoring and weighing in at Herbal Magic three times a week. I was accountable to someone; they were keeping score.

What I liked most about the program was that it allowed me to pick the foods I enjoyed and buy them at my local supermarket. I eliminated sugar, salt, and fried foods from my diet completely, and I stopped buying anything that was prepackaged and processed.

I haven't eaten pizza in three years. Pizza is my trigger food. If I start, I can't stop, so I avoid it entirely.

MY FITNESS PROGRAM

I was seven months into the weight-loss program when I joined the fitness club. At first it was a challenge to make the time and put in the effort, but now I go five times a week.

Six months into the fitness routine, though, I wasn't seeing the results I had expected. Then I began working out with Mike Clements, a professional bodybuilder and personal trainer. Because I have a torn meniscus (a common knee injury), Clements customized a safe, results-oriented program for me. With every workout, he watched my form and pushed me to the limit — beyond what I had done on my own.

After three years of staying focused on my goal — regaining my health and becoming more fit — I have lost 50 inches and nearly 50 pounds. I celebrated my 50th birthday dancing the rumba in the arms of my devoted husband, Michael. I've changed my wardrobe entirely. I wear dresses and skirts that complement my figure and I feel like a woman again. And I have resumed wearing heels.

When I was overweight I felt invisible. Now I feel brand new and ready to enjoy another 50 years.

WHAT I LEARNED
Don't kid yourself that you can lose weight and then go back to your old eating habits. Losing weight and keeping it off is a lifestyle change, not a short-term application.

MORNING STARTER
I like to start my day with Agnes Ramsay's recipe for Baked Apple Oatmeal — it sticks to my ribs and sustains me all morning. It is made with egg whites, grated apple, and skim milk, plus a few other ingredients. I top it with fresh or frozen blueberries and sugar-free apple jam. For the full recipe, visit activeadultmag.com. Ramsay is a personal trainer (agnes9@sympatico.ca).

AFTER WORKOUT NUTRITION
I enjoy either of these "power" beverages after a workout.

- vanilla bean ISO protein shake with 8 ounces of Bolthouse Farms 50/50 Berry (fruit and vegetable blend)
- VegeGreens mixed with 4 ounces of cherry juice and 4 ounces of water

Foods like fruits and veggies that are rich in nutrients work best to sustain me between meals.

ON OCCASION

I still crave chocolate once in a while but limit myself to one Dove Dark Chocolate Square. Honestly, I can actually eat just one. Each square has 40 calories and 2.5 grams of fat.

A SOURCE OF INSPIRATION

I look forward to each issue of *Clean Eating* magazine. Each issue includes a success story, fitness routines, and lots of mouth-watering, super-low-fat recipes. I also refer to these companion books: *The Eat-Clean Diet* and *The Eat-Clean Diet Workout* by Tosca Reno, published by Robert Kennedy Publishing. To learn more about clean eating, visit www.eatcleandiet.com.

MAUREEN CATANIA'S 10 TIPS FOR HEALTHY EATING

1. Eliminate all trigger foods from your diet.
2. Develop simple, positive behaviors that will support the new you.
3. If you are physically capable, commit to a fitness routine.
4. Seek a weight-loss program to suit your needs.
5. Join a busy gym. It will motivate you to work out.
6. If you slip up, don't get discouraged. Get help.
7. Forecast attainable short-term goals.
8. Reward good results with something other than food.
9. Throw out your "fat" clothes and invest in something new.
10. Change your attitude and you will change your life.

JOURNALING WITH LESLEY SHORE

"My chief want in life is someone who shall make me do what I can."
–Ralph Waldo Emerson

Thursday mornings I manage two hours of exercise. For me, a life-long couch potato, that's amazing. One day in my mailbox I found a flyer about an exercise class that takes place in the party room of my condo for one hour. I walk the ravine for 45 minutes first and then do the class for an hour.

In my early 60s I'm the youngest participant. Most of the others are in their 70s and 80s and many are in their 90s. They've had their share of health issues and heartbreak. But Thursday morning at 10, there they are in their fitness gear ready to pump it up for a full hour. If you think Audrey, the teacher, lets us off easy, you're mistaken. Her routine is as challenging as the ones on the DVDs I'm using.

"You can improve your balance, you know," Audrey shouts out to us regularly.

And guess what? She's right. The people in my exercise class keep me real, inspire me, and show me the power of exercise.

START JOURNALING

Where are you with your accountability network? Have you found a fitness buddy or joined an online network? Write in your FIT Journal for 20 minutes about the steps you've taken or plan to take. If it helps, set your timer again.

Here are some topics you can write about: Who is going to pace you on your journey? What have you noticed in reading this chapter that you didn't expect? What obstacles have you discovered to making progress? What has surprised you? Have any new goals or dreams surfaced? How are you feeling about your body and yourself today?

Power Source Tool #4

Define Success and Set Goals

"Goals are dreams with deadlines."

–STEPHEN GRELLET

The first step toward having unstoppable motivation — a key element of, and result of, mental fitness — is to determine your goals.

But before you determine your goals, it's important for you to have a basic understanding of the psychology of goal setting.

Studies have shown that people who set clear decisive goals are more likely to achieve what they have set out to do and as a result have a higher success rate. If you set out to start exercising without setting specific goals, chances are you will find yourself directionless at times and at a greater risk of giving up.

The process of sitting down and mapping out your fitness goals is a powerful technique. You will be designing a plan that provides you with direction; this will help you to stay focused. It's important to have a vision of what you want to achieve. It's okay to dream about how you want to feel and look physically, but to actualize those dreams you're going to need specific and realistic goals.

Another important point to consider when defining your fitness goals is to take your big goals and break them down into smaller, more easily achievable, short-term goals. Smaller goals that lead to a bigger goal are less threatening. They therefore improve your success rate.

For example, if your long-term goal is to run in a 10-mile charitable event at the end of the summer, then you can break that challenge into two training stages. Stage one is to train toward running five miles within one month. Stage two is to run the ten miles by the end of the second month. This is a strategy that sets you up for success.

The idea is to set good goals: ones that are important to you, tell you where you are going, and show how far you have yet to go. The secret is to align your goals with your basic values.

Here are a few pointers to follow:

1. Write down your fitness/health goals.
2. Specify a completion date for your big goals.
3. Break down your big goals into smaller goals and indicate dates by which they will be achieved.
4 Define obstacles and find ways to overcome them.
5. Define how you're going to reward yourself as you achieve your goals.
6. Visualize achieving your goals.

As you begin your fitness program, you can decide on the ways in which you will measure success. Success is not always measured in the pounds and inches you lose. It may be measured in strength, endurance, and even time and duration.

Susan's Story

To set realistic short-term and long-term goals for both of the marathons I completed, I started by assessing my strengths and weaknesses. I knew it would take me seven and a half hours to complete the marathons, that the streets would be reopened by the time I came in, and that I might be the last person to finish (I *was* in my second marathon). I knew I would never be able to compete with anyone else during the races. While I realized I would not have speed, I knew I *did* have stamina and resilience.

My training goals for the marathons included: training for seven months; completing the training and the marathons without injury; having peaceful mornings, gorgeous routes, and stress-free walks and jogs; and cross-training with weights, Cycle Fit classes, stretching, and core conditioning. My long-term goal is to continue to do weight and strength training so I can complete three half-marathons every year.

Some mornings my only goal was to get up, get dressed, and get out the door.

Theresa's Story

My short-term goals, as I prepared for my training for two marathons in the summer of 2010 and fall of 2010 *and* planned my return to judo (my second favorite sport) in 2010, were to design and follow an optimal nutritional and training program to build up my immune system and physical strength.

My long-term goals? To join a cycling team in the summer and begin riding outdoors, and to continue my fitness leadership pursuit by training to be an aerobics dance instructor later in the year.

SEVEN STRATEGIES FOR DEFINING SUCCESS AND SETTING GOALS

#1. Believe in yourself and your ability to achieve success
Look at the goals you have already accomplished in your life. Note that you are already successful. Aim high. Focus your energy, reduce distractions, and find new ways to achieve your goals. Above all, visualize your body and feel the energy.

#2. Be gentle with yourself

Maintain a positive mental attitude. Find ways to celebrate when you achieve a goal and watch your enthusiasm increase and your confidence soar. Avoid comparing yourself with other people and their accomplishments.

#3. Set S.M.A.R.T. goals

   S = Specific

   M = Measurable

   A = Attainable: goals you can achieve

   R = Realistic: based on your body, health restrictions, etc.

   T = Timely: specific dates written in your FIT Action Plan (see the chapter *Power Source Tool #7*)

Break your goals into steps. Short-term goals give you milestones for staying sharp and motivated throughout the journey. They also help you to deal with setbacks and fluctuations.

#4. Don't try to do too much, too soon

Just because you rode a bicycle when you were a child doesn't mean you should enter a cycling race. Be realistic about what your body can achieve.

#5. At the same time, set bigger goals and blue-sky goals

Keep an eye on the distant goal and you will steadily improve on the way to achieving it. Look at where you want to be in six months, a year, two years, and five years. For example, break down the training for a 10k run or walk into the number of miles or kilometers per day, week, and month.

Blue-sky goals challenge you to ignite the great potential that lies within you — to become the person you were meant to be. Here are some to think about:

- A marathon
- A triathlon
- A cycling race
- A masters competition
- A swimming competition

#6. Be energized by the progress you make toward your fitness goals

Be patient with yourself. It may take time to see the results, but as time progresses, you will be advancing toward your goals.

#7. Keep track of your progress in your Power Source Weekly FIT Training Log

At the end of the chapter *Power Source Tool #7* later in this book, we have created a Weekly FIT Training Log that you can use to track your progress on a daily, weekly, and monthly basis. We include some sample entries from Dorina Vendramin`s Weekly FIT Training Log.

Unless you write down and track your goals, they are likely to get lost in the shuffle and excitement of new problems, new challenges, and new decisions.

Chart your progress and make adjustments to your goals and plan.

Create a giant calendar with workouts indicated; add a smiley-face sticker for each workout you do. Post this calendar in a prominent place.

OUR POWER SOURCE EXPERT, RUTH KRONGOLD, SPEAKS

I hope to continue with my present fitness activities while incorporating more stretching for easing arthritic stiffness and adding weights for strength. As well, I hope to remain vital and active as I age, knowing that vulnerability and weakness are the flip side of strength.

OUR POWER SOURCE WOMEN SPEAK

We asked our Power Source Women about their fitness goals and how they define success.

Audrey

It is more difficult to define goals and success in group fitness. There is no time to match or distance to complete.

I work as hard as I can at every class and some days I do better than others. A class that may have seemed hard a few months ago may be easier now.

For some types of classes, like boxing, mastering the techniques is a goal in itself. On a recent week-long ski trip in the Alps, my legs didn't hurt as much and I didn't feel the altitude as much because I had prepared for this activity by changing some of my classes prior to the trip.

Edna

My fitness goals and objectives are to keep going. Since I became a personal trainer at age 65, I appreciate how fortunate I am to be so fit and have a body that works. My short-term and long-term goals are identical: to keep my body moving and continue to build muscle strength and endurance. It's the only way.

Pat

Originally my goal was to complete a marathon without an injury and enjoy the experience. I completed two Ottawa Marathons, needing recovery time only for sore toes. Another goal is to be consistent with exercise.

Phyllis

I would like to train to teach a muscle-works class. I enjoy instructing classes and this is one class that would be a good challenge for me and something to work toward.

OUR ROLE MODEL #3: ABBEY SMITH

MY STORY

Born in the 1940s I had a typical middle-class-girl's upbringing, the aim of which was to protect me and to make me marriageable. Traditional power imbalances, based on gender, reigned in my family and school environment. At school, I was always the smallest in any class or on any team. My mom sent me to ballet lessons, where my flexibility and enthusiasm helped me. However, for decades I had anger-management issues and a feeling of being at a disadvantage.

When I became an adult and had my own family responsibilities, it was clear to me that to be effective in caring for others I had to take good care of myself first. I began to embrace physical activities, as long as they were enjoyable.

I started in an unusual women's dance class, learned some yoga, and at the age of 40 began jogging and running. I felt a great sense of freedom speeding along a path under my own power, and I learned about my breathing and how it responded to activity.

MY WAKE-UP CALL

The women's dance class I attended, which began in the 1970s under Doris Mehegan's formidable leadership, was empowering. We challenged our abilities and the limits of balance, strength, expression, cooperation, and trust. I learned there is a kind of memory in the body.

Later, when I attended a very challenging class in Iyengar yoga, my ability to learn and to meet the uncomfortable demands of the practice was a revelation to me.

In my 50s, when my adolescent daughter told me there was "nothing I could do" to keep her off the streets at night, I enrolled us together in a women's self-defense class where we practiced awareness, alertness, and defensive actions.

It was there that I first heard about Aikido, from the course leader, Fran Turner, and her two male assistants. It is a Japanese martial art for self-defense that takes the energy of the attacker and turns it back onto the attacker, leaving him or her unharmed.

The Japanese word *Aikido* is written with three characters that translate as "the Way of Spiritual Harmony." Harmonious movement, or blending, is shaped by a philosophy of harmony. There are no competitions or tournaments in Aikido. Emphasis is on self-mastery, not on controlling others. Rank is awarded by a testing procedure that demonstrates student growth. Regular and frequent practice develops skills through constant repetition of techniques.

Movements in Aikido may be spectacular and send the attacker flying, or they may be small and control the wrist and elbow joints in subtle but persuasive ways.

MY SOLUTION

Fran Sensei, a powerful, small woman who was in her 50s at the time, inspired me to attend her classes in Aikido. I started to practice this martial art for physical fitness and for self-defense, and because I was fascinated by its non-violent philosophy. In time, as I continued to practice, I started to really enjoy myself.

MY FITNESS PROGRAM

Now, I practice at least three times a week, in the evenings and on Saturday mornings.

On Sunday mornings I take a Stott Pilates class. It helps with my case of pelvic organ prolapse, which was diagnosed four years ago.

At the age of 67, after 12 years of slow learning, I agreed to present myself for testing to receive my first-degree black belt in Aikido (*Shodan*). Preparing for that event was more psychologically than physically challenging. I went to the *dojo* (practice space) six or seven days a week for three months to practice the techniques and focus my attention. My teachers and all the other students were rooting for me.

After 15 years of practice, I am the oldest female member of Shugyo Dojo Toronto, a non-profit organization. I enjoy teaching workshops and a children's class and supporting my fellow students.

Being small is not really a problem for me; in fact, it is an advantage in Aikido, which does not rely on size or strength for its effectiveness. Best of all, there are no winners or losers in Aikido. Every participant benefits.

What I also learned is that I enjoy the power that Aikido techniques allow. My acquired fears of larger, stronger men gradually evaporated, and I became patient with myself and my limitations.

I do not learn as quickly as I did when I was younger, and I still need encouragement from a strong teacher. Without doubt, maintaining fitness will always be a goal for me.

ABBEY SMITH'S TIPS FOR HARMONIZING YOUR BODY, MIND, AND SPIRIT

1. Training in Aikido enables the student to encounter stressful circumstances without being thrown off-kilter.
2. It also creates a resiliency of body and openness of mind — qualities needed in society and in our daily lives.

JOURNALING WITH LESLEY SHORE

"Life begins at the end of your comfort zone." –Neale Donald Walsch

Last year my son invited me to visit him in Melbourne, Australia, where he was then working. He'd take some time off work and we would travel to Sydney and other tourist spots. I booked my flights, thrilled to visit a country I'd wanted to see since I was a kid.

One evening he called.

"Mom, I want you to go onto the website www.bridgewalk.com," he said.

"Why?" I asked.

"Because it describes one of the best things to do in Sydney and I would love to do it with you."

The bridge walk takes place on the famous Sydney Harbour Bridge: the one beside the magnificent Opera House. You actually walk up to the very top of the arched bridge span and then along it. The panorama of Sydney is below you.

But I'm terrified of heights.

There I was, torn between wanting to please my son — because nothing athletic frightens him — and my own desperate fear. I vacillated. Three days before we were due to arrive in Sydney, I knew we had to make our reservations. We did. I hardly slept the night before the walk.

We were fortunate to wake up to a bright, sunny, clear morning with little wind. When the group leader asked each participant why we were there, I shot my hand up.

"I'm here because I was intimidated into it. I'm terrified of heights."

"That's no problem," he said. "We've had lots of people like you do this. I'll be here for you."

Guess what? I did it. It will remain one of the proudest moments of my life.

Jot down in your FIT Journal the topics in this chapter that appealed to you. Which are not your style? Each of us nurtures a secret dream, something we'd love to do but don't think we're capable of. What we don't realize is that we're our own worst enemies, holding ourselves back from giving it the old college try.

Write about your private dream. Your goal. What limits would you like to push yourself beyond? How much determination do you think you can bring to realizing it? Do you believe you can go the distance? If not, why not?

Set the timer again and let your thoughts run free.

Power Source Tool #5

Create Fitness Routines Aligned with Your Goals

"Motivation is what gets you started.
Habit is what keeps you going."

–JIM RYUN

Most people have started a fitness program more than once. It may be hard for them to stick to their program for a variety of reasons: they lose their energy and enthusiasm, they get distracted by other things, or they don't see results quickly enough.

Creating lifetime fitness habits can seem like an impossible task, requiring significant time and effort. The thought of fitting something else into an already crowded life seems impossible to many. Yet fitness is about patience, persistence, and maintaining good habits. It is a way of life.

What motivates people to break old habits, create new routines, and stay focused? To no sooner skip their regular workout than go without brushing their teeth?

This final chapter on mental fitness shows how you can make fitness a life-long habit. The habits you develop determine your health. The simple things you do on a daily basis can lead you to disease or to a sense of well-being and longevity. The direction you take depends on the way you use your power source within to choose.

Susan's Story

I used to snack on crackers and cookies throughout the day — a handful here and another handful there. For as long as I can remember, I drank Diet Coke as a way to control my weight. These two habits, combined with smoking, were part of my life for 25 years.

In 1980 I stopped smoking cold turkey. Fifteen years later I stopped drinking diet soft drinks. And finally, about five years ago, I started to consciously think about eating simply and sensibly and to cut out mindless snacking.

I started by getting rid of the crackers I kept in my house — they were my trigger food. I concentrated on having three meals and two healthy snacks each day. Today, I am 20 pounds lighter. I make sure I always have nuts, apples, and oranges as snacks in my purse, desk, and car. I drink lots of water. And I still indulge in small portions of the things I enjoy, such as chocolates and ice cream.

In order to work out in the morning, I changed my sleeping habits. I am now asleep early most nights (unless I am teaching or out for dinner), up at 4:30 a.m., and at the gym by 5:30 a.m. That schedule won't work for everyone, but it's the best solution for me.

And I always leave my gym clothes *and* my clothes for the next day in the hallway the night before. In the morning before I go to the gym I put on everything I will wear that day. That way I don't forget socks or underwear or pack two different colored shoes (all of which I have done in the past).

Theresa's Story

Missing lunch during busy clinical days was wreaking havoc with my energy level and was incompatible with my beliefs about health. I found it a challenge to find time during the day to have proper meals. I needed to address this problem — and address it fast.

My new routines involve ensuring that I have plenty of nutritious foods that do not require cooking. I take the time each day to prepare power salads that consist of every food group and lots of essential vitamins. Also, I make sure I am well stocked with snacks like nuts, seeds, fruits, and rice cakes so a supply of good calories is immediately available to me when I feel hungry. Most importantly I keep water by my side at all times.

SEVEN STRATEGIES FOR BREAKING HABITS AND CREATING NEW ROUTINES

#1. Define the habits that interfere with your fitness goals
Then analyze what would motivate you to give up, reduce, or eliminate those habits in order to achieve your fitness goals.

#2. What would you gain by changing these habits?
Your answer could be that you would feel fit, increase your sense of well-being, have more energy, reduce your stress and/or depression, sleep more soundly, be alert and relaxed, manage your weight, or look better.

#3. Describe the new routines you want to incorporate into your life and how you can make these changes
What changes can you start with? What can you substitute for your unwanted thoughts, feelings, or behaviors?
   Suggestions include:
   • Arrange a weekly meal plan that includes natural, healthy foods.
   • Get more sleep so your muscles can repair and grow.

- Go to the gym or work out at home, instead of thinking about it.
- Develop more challenging cardio workouts or use heavier weights.

#4. Develop daily rituals to help you
- Put your workout clothes on top of your dresser or by the door.
- Park your running shoes right next to the bed, unlaced, so all you have to do is step into them and you're ready to go.
- Pack your gym bag, prepare meals and snacks, and plan what you'll do that day.
- Keep a full water bottle in the refrigerator.
- Have an exercise video ready to go when you get home at night.

5. Select the time of day that works best for your workouts based on your lifestyle
Develop a plan to incorporate fitness into your daily routines.

Morning:
- Before you jump into the shower, do a few sets of push-ups, crunches, and squats.
- Fit a few stretches or sit-ups in while waiting for your morning coffee to brew.
- Hop onto the treadmill or stationary bicycle while you listen to the radio, watch the morning news, or relax with your iPod.
- Step outside for a brisk walk.
- Allow yourself enough time to eat something light

before you hit the gym or start to exercise. Exercising on an empty stomach will cause your body to break down muscle in order to have enough energy. Once you've adjusted to early-morning workouts, add to the routine.

- Play a game of golf before heading off to work.
- Swim early in the morning, when the pool is not as busy.

Lunchtime:

- Whether you eat lunch at home or at work, take a break and devote the time to you.
- Bring a comfortable pair of walking shoes to work with you. Go for a short walk with colleagues or drive to a nearby mall and walk.
- Join a gym and attend a noon-hour class. Shower and enjoy the second half of your day.

Throughout the day:

- Ride a bicycle to and from work, on errands, or along trails. **G**
- Get off the subway, streetcar, or bus several stops before your destination and walk to work, or park at the farthest end of a parking lot. **G**
- Do errands on foot instead of by car. **G**
- Take hills instead of going around them. **G**

At home:

- Squeeze in a few ten-minute walks throughout the day. If you don't have time for a full workout, recognize the value of shorter spurts of exercise spaced throughout the day.

- Wear your workout clothes during the day. This gets you in the mood to move.
- Take the stairs in your apartment building instead of the elevator, and go and up and down several times a day. Walk back and forth in the hallways of your apartment building or home. ❂

At work:
- Take walking breaks throughout the day.
- Put a pair of hand-grippers in your drawer. These provide a great finger and forearm workout for when you're on long conference calls or between e-mails.
- If your commute involves riding the bus or train or you drive and often have to sit in stalled traffic, take along and use a pair of hand-grippers.

After work:
- Go to the gym on your way home.

Evenings:
- Evenings are a great opportunity for some quick calisthenics. Do some basic exercises for 10 to 20 minutes, such as jumping jacks, stretches, jogging on the spot, jumping rope, sit-ups, and sets of crunches. Consider lifting dumbbells during television commercials.
- If you are a night owl, try not to exercise too late. Working out too close to bedtime, such as an hour or so before you go to sleep, will disrupt your sleep.

On weekends:
- Set the clock early and go for a walk or run while you have the world to yourself.

- Rethink your weekend rituals. Try a Saturday bike ride, a rock-climbing lesson, or a swim in a pool.
- Look for scenic routes for weekly walks and bike rides with your family, friends, or alone — all year round. ✹Ⓖ
- Wash your car by hand. ✹Ⓖ
- Get rid of labor-saving devices such as snow blowers and electric lawn mowers. Get out your shovel or push mower and use your own energy for these tasks. ✹Ⓖ

#6. Commit to our Functional FIT Workout Plan.
- See the chapter *Power Source Tool #7* for our Functional FIT Workout Plan that you can do at home.

#7. Assess progress flowing from your new routines. Check off the items that apply:
- You are getting a good night's sleep.
- Your clothes fit better.
- You think more clearly.
- You have more energy.
- You can lift heavier weights.
- You can work out longer without feeling exhausted.
- You notice your resting heart rate drop over time.
- You hear your doctor congratulate you on your improved health.

OUR POWER SOURCE EXPERT, RUTH KRONGOLD, SPEAKS

I have broken the habit of thinking of myself as uncoordinated. Daily fitness activities are now habitual and help me to resist the urge to think poorly of myself physically or emotionally.

During my 20s I gave up meat, alcohol, and smoking. I have replaced these habits with a fairly healthy diet (including occasional chocolate binges). I still struggle with the habit of worrying.

OUR POWER SOURCE WOMEN SPEAK

We asked our Power Source Women to describe the habits they have broken as well as the new fitness routines they have created. We asked them about the habits they found particularly difficult to change.

Audrey

None of us likes to do what we're not good at. But I've learned to keep an open mind. I will try just about any group fitness activity at least once — outdoor boot camp, hip-hop, fencing, cardio salsa, and hot yoga are a few examples of things that haven't worked out long-term for me. There was a time when I worked out seven days a week and freaked if I missed a workout. Now I consider fitness a lifetime pursuit. I take breaks if I need to or want to.

I intentionally leave some components out of my fitness routine. I do weight (sculpt) classes but these are mostly endurance weights with light dumbbells. Classes don't really afford a good opportunity to do real strength training with heavier weights. I seldom go into the weight room to do weights by myself. And although stretching is a part of every aerobics class and my one yoga class a week also involves a fair bit of stretching, I seldom add extra stretching to my routine.

Edna

The one nasty habit I succeeded in breaking was my continuous dieting — how liberating it is to be rid of that one! New habits that I have created include healthy eating, getting to bed earlier, and a promise to myself that I will continue to exercise forevermore. Habits I could not change? My inability to relax. My need and greed to experience as much as possible of life — all the time — which sometimes results in a frenetic lifestyle.

Pat

For the past 30 years I have had a habit of working out first thing in the morning, at 5:30. As a result I am more conscious of my body and I eat healthier.

I have also been working hard to do more things for myself instead of always doing things for others.

Phyllis

Today I am more aware of my body. Although I would still like to lose some weight, I know what it takes to do that and my plan is a healthy one. I still have the occasional trigger, but exercise helps me tremendously as I strive toward a fitter me.

JOURNALING WITH LESLEY SHORE

"Life brings you opportunities and we do our best to avoid them! Go with life instead." –Paul Lowe

I have a great procrastination routine: wake up, make the bed, check my e-mail, empty the dishwasher, water the plants, fold the laundry, and throw in a new load. By then the phone starts ringing and I answer, knowing full well that if I don't get to my exercising before 10, I'll have to skip it for the day. Yet all I have to do is pull on some tights and a T-shirt, do up my runners, and step outside the door. The ravine is right there waiting for me. All 45 glorious minutes of it.

But I am improving. Because the exercise is a reward in itself. I feel better on the days I exercise and that motivates me to want to do it more than to empty the dishwasher, fold the laundry, etc., which I've been doing religiously for years without any benefit whatsoever to my well-being. It takes 30 days to make a new habit. Then you find you can't live without it. You feel out of sorts, not yourself. You wonder why you're having a bad day.

START JOURNALING

Are you a procrastinator or a take-charge person? What will help keep you faithful to the changes you want to make? What bad habits have you broken already in the past? Which ones do you still need to break? What could trip you up and how will you get around those demons? Open up your FIT Journal, set the timer for 20 minutes again, and let go.

PART 2

Physical Fitness: Change Your Body

Power Source Tool #6

Discover Your FIT
Motivational Style™

"People often say that motivation doesn't last.
Well, neither does bathing —
that's why we recommend it daily."

–ZIG ZIGLAR

It's time for you to focus more closely on physical fitness, the subject of the second part of this book. Now that you know how important changing your mind is to changing your body, you need to determine the type of physical fitness program that best fits who you are and what your needs are. This chapter will help you to determine your motivational style and the fitness activities and approaches that best fit that style.

GETTING MOTIVATED

Motivation can be thought of as the energy and drive to learn, work effectively, and achieve the goals you set for yourself.

The following exercise will help you get started on the hunt for your motivational style.

A Visualization Exercise

Take a moment to imagine how you would feel *after* a great workout.

Find a quiet place and reflect on the physical satisfaction as well as the feeling of accomplishment. Feel how relaxed you are and notice how your face shines after that good workout. You feel energized and focused, ready to take on any challenge.

Now bring to mind the aspects of exercise you dislike. What is your biggest reason for avoiding exercise? Are you too tired? Do you not have enough time? Is physical exertion too much of a hassle? Pinpoint your greatest complaint about exercise.

Now hold these two images of exercise in your mind and complete the following task.

Draw up the image of your exercise complaint in your mind. The image is likely to be clear and accompanied by sounds, smells, and sensations. Capture all of this through this exercise. In your mind slowly begin to fade this picture to black and white and distance the image until it is dull, fuzzy, and remote.

Draw the image of the wonderful feeling you would have after accomplishing a great workout. Magnify this image in your mind. Concentrate on how you feel physically, mentally, and emotionally. View the experience in bright colors and add a sound track of inspirational music.

Did you know that music is a great motivator? Many people find relief and pleasure with music. Try some mystical Enigma or soothing Brahms. Whatever your pleasure, add some beautiful music to your visualization to enhance your motivation and get you excited about exercise.

INSPIRATION, ASPIRATION, PERSPIRATION

INSPIRATION

People can be a source of inspiration. That's why this book is full of stories of women who at one point or another overcame a challenging obstacle by finding a fitness passion and refocusing their energy. Seek inspiration from these women and use their stories to help you develop your own.

ASPIRATION

We all have dreams and goals we want to achieve in our lives. Think about what you aspire to be, experience, or have. Now consider how being fit will help you to get there.

PERSPIRATION

There may be times when the challenge of adhering to an exercise program to achieve your new fitness goals becomes overwhelming. There may be times when you hit a few roadblocks along the way. By focusing on progress rather than perfection, you can start each day with continuing determination. The key is to never stop trying.

Finding your fitness passion and building your health can be an exciting journey. Remember to focus on today and believe that each moment is taking you closer to your special relationship with fitness.

THE IMPORTANCE OF MOTIVATION

Motivation is possibly the biggest determining factor when it comes to creating and implementing fitness in your life. Your level of motivation can make or break your program.

It is crucial for you, before beginning your fitness program, to be clear about your underlying values and feelings about the goals you are setting. If you are clear and you feel 100 percent committed to achieving them, it will be easier for you to stay on track and not allow things to hinder your success.

There will be times when you feel tired and are just not in the mood. When that happens, you're going to need the support of both intrinsic and extrinsic motivators to keep you in the game.

By reflecting on how good you would feel after a workout, you are activating your intrinsic motivation. That means you are generating positive thoughts of the benefits associated with exercising, thoughts that can help keep you on track. But when that isn't enough to keep you in the fitness game, you may need extrinsic motivating rewards. For example, you could pull out a pair of slacks that you once fit into and set a date in the near future to be wearing them again. This is a sure way to add a little spark to your motivation and keep you on track with your fitness goal.

INTRODUCING OUR FIT MOTIVATIONAL STYLE QUESTIONNAIRE™

You are about to complete a questionnaire to help you define the environment that will be most conducive to your exercise success. The FIT Motivational Style Questionnaire™ captures two dimensions that are important for exercise success: the *social* and the *competitive*. Your FIT Motivational Style™ will be based on the degree to which you are motivated by social participation and competitiveness. For example, the style called "Creative Designer" fits someone who enjoys group participation because it naturally motivates them and gives them structure. This individual is high in the social dimension but low in competitiveness.

FIT Motivational Styles should be understood as *trends* in a person's orientation. The styles are not static but help an individual to get the fitness process going. These styles may evolve as a person's fitness increases. A person could even move into another style category.

Now it's time for you to complete the questionnaire. Once you have filled it out and scored it (see the scoring instructions following the questionnaire), you will know your FIT Motivational Style™. We will show you how this will help you to determine the activities that best fit your style — and therefore the FIT environment that is right for you.

Our FIT Motivational Style Questionnaire™

The following statements involve a variety of situations related to fitness. Read each one carefully and circle the response that best describes what your feelings and attitudes would be if you were in that particular situation.

1. *Today you plan to have a serious workout. You will exercise:*
    1. Alone and at your own pace.
    2. With a friend.
    3. With a team or group.
    4. Following your training plan.

2. *It's Sunday night and you are thinking about your workouts for the week. You:*
    1. Plan what you are going to do ahead of time.
    2. Get to the gym and find out what class you can participate in.
    3. Meet a friend or a group for a morning run/walk.
    4. Go to the gym, get on a treadmill, and push yourself. It's Monday and you want a great start to your week.

3. *You have just moved into your new home and you are excited because of the great park that is nearby. You have been anticipating the invigorating walks you will take there each day. Just as you're leaving for your first walk, a few family members show up. What do you do?*
    1. Pass on going. Say to yourself you'll do it another time when you have no distractions.
    2. Decide there's no rush for the walk. You'll go later that day when time permits.

3. Tell your family members you were on your way out for a walk and invite them to join you.
4. As soon as they leave, put on your runners and hit the park with the intention of extending your walk to make up for the slack.

4. You've just joined a new gym and your plan is to get into better shape. What type of training will you probably go with?
1. Ask for a personal trainer to give you a program and work with the individual for a few sessions.
2. Hit the conditioning area and start pumping some iron. You've done this before so you can figure it out or you'll ask someone.
3. Check out the class schedule and plan on taking a few classes each week.
4. Find out if they have any groups that are training, such as running groups, swimming groups, etc.

5. A 5k walk is being held just blocks away from your house on Sunday. The money raised from the registrations is going to a charitable cause. You decide to:
1. Skip it and follow your program at home or at the gym.
2. Walk over and join in with the spectators to cheer the crowd on.
3. Call up your friend and ask him or her to join you in the walk.
4. Sign up and try to challenge yourself by walking the route in the shortest time.

6. *You were planning on working out at the end of the day but are stressed out. You:*

1. Continue with what needs to get done and plan to work out tomorrow.
2. Grab a good self-help book, make yourself a cup of tea, and read.
3. Go to a coffee shop nearby with a friend to chat and then maybe go for the walk together afterwards.
4. Go for a brisk walk or hit the gym anyway and work the stress out.

7. *You are in a fitness class you are quite familiar with. Suddenly, the instructor has to leave and asks you to take over the last half of the class. You:*

1. Say you need a little training first, but would like to do it next time. Suggest he or she ask someone else.
2. Agree to take over and try to recall what you have been taught so it's close to the usual class, plus add a few things you think of along the way.
3. Jump in, grab the microphone, and wing it the best you can.
4. Think of this as an opportunity to motivate the group and be seen as a leader.

8. *You arrive at the pool to swim and all of the lanes are busy. You certainly could squeeze your way in, but after evaluating the pool you decide to:*

1. Check with the lifeguard for the days and times the pool isn't so busy and plan to return on one of those days.
2. Go to the conditioning area and work out with weights.

3. Get in the pool and just do your best to swim with the crowd.
4. Swim in the lane that looks like it has the more serious swimmers and less splashing.

9. *The yoga class you decide to try turns out to be too advanced for you. You decide to:*
   1. Find another class better suited to your level.
   2. Tell the instructor you are new and need help with the different moves in the class.
   3. Put your mat next to a friendly face or two and try to follow what they are doing.
   4. Challenge yourself and try the moves.

10. *You have been following a training plan to participate in your first 25k charitable bike race. The day of the race you are not feeling at your best. You:*
   1. Decide to pass on it and sign up for another race in the near future. This way you can keep your training up to speed.
   2. Put together a care package with a few things you think you may need along the way, e.g., protein bar, aspirin, etc.
   3. Go anyway, just taking it easy and staying close to the group of friends you know at the race — letting them know how you're feeling.
   4. Tell yourself you'll feel better after the race. You would be more disappointed if you didn't attempt to complete the race.

YOUR FIT MOTIVATIONAL STYLE™ IS ...

SELF-DIRECTED SOLOIST

If you scored **10–17** points you are a *Self-Directed Soloist*, the power-from-within type.

You prefer to plan out your daily workout schedule. You are self-reliant. Your self-energized style makes it easy for you to go solo when it comes to your fitness. You are reasonably comfortable when faced with a sudden change in your planned workout schedule, and your ability to be flexible allows you to make a quick decision on how you will alter your exercise plans. Setbacks are expected. You recognize that they do not mean you cannot achieve your fitness goals.

Exercises that allow you the opportunity to improve at your own pace suit you best. However, you may enjoy hiring a personal trainer to work with you to map out a detailed plan so when you go it alone there is more structure to your workout.

Your strong inner drive keeps you persevering to meet your fitness goals regardless of what gets in the way and how long it takes.

FIT Reinforcers for the Self-Directed Soloist: Keep a journal of what you are doing, or, even better, put up a cork or vinyl board and track your workouts so you can see how you are doing whenever you pass by. Give yourself a pat on the back for sticking to your program.

FIT Detractors for the Self-Directed Soloist: Because you are self-motivated and stick to your own agenda, you probably like routine and habituate pretty quickly once you find something that works. You could run into the rigidity zone, so make it a point to review your plan at least once a month to see how you might tweak it and add some new zest. Don't get stuck in a pattern.

FIT Activities for the Self-Directed Soloist: gardening, home training videos, horseback riding, ice-skating, indoor/outdoor cycling, in-line skating, jogging, mini-trampoline, swimming, walking, weight training, and yoga.

CREATIVE DESIGNER

If you scored **18–24** points you are a *Creative Designer*, the light, energized type.

You are motivated by an environment that is light and fun. You like to get inspired watching others get into action. But you are also the type of person who has the ability to inspire others because of your relaxed, uplifting spirit. You can be playful yet are often firm and dedicated in the challenges you take on.

You have great energy potential, but the occasional quieting of your mind is essential when your creative juices become exhausted. You have the ability to focus your energy with concentration combined with enthusiasm and freshness. When you are turned on by a particular type of exercise, you can be passionate and hot; but if there is no turn-on, then the energy slows down and things get cold. At that point, you lose interest in the particular activity and need to move on.

Your fit is with dance classes, aerobics, or any class that is interesting and has lots of energy to keep your mind activated and your body moving. You may enjoy activities where there is more of a social component and freedom to move around. You don't mind a schedule set out for you when attending a class, but sometimes you might like to hit the gym and just do whatever comes to mind that day.

FIT Reinforcers for the Creative Designer: Displaying a visual that maps out how you are doing with your fitness goals can be quite a motivator. Use a cork or bristol board for this project. Design a one-month calendar to document your workouts. Make it attractive by cutting out colorful uplifting pictures of health and fitness from different magazines. Paste or tape them onto your board to add a little pizzazz to your calendar.

Now hang it up so you see it each day and start to track your progress. Make sure you have some colorful markers nearby for marking your daily workouts. This will be a sure way of energizing that creative designer within you and inspiring you to keep moving toward your fitness goals.

FIT Detractors for the Creative Designer: Because you are light in nature and your environment can have a major influence on the way you feel and on your exercise, make sure you stay away from environments that generate low energy. Connect with people and spaces that add to your enthusiasm, i.e., with people who have a similar uplifting spirit. This will help you succeed in your fitness pursuit.

FIT Activities for the Creative Designer: high/low impact aerobic classes, baseball, basketball, curling, folk dancing, frisbee, indoor/outdoor cycling, Pilates, running (with a partner or group), square dancing, tai chi, volleyball, weight training, in a muscle works class, water aerobics, yoga.

SPIRITED PLANNER

If you scored **25–31** points you are a *Spirited Planner*, the self-disciplined social type.

You are motivated by self-discipline. You like to adhere to structure, but you also enjoy the social component on occasion in your activities.

Nature has given you a sophisticated guidance system in your feelings. You have developed an awareness of your emotions, which guides you when you're structuring your daily activities.

You also have an adventurous side that comes out in your physical strength, and that is why you are usually open to taking on a new challenge when it comes your way. You may prefer the outdoors so you can participate in a natural environment. You try to remain energetic, lively, and optimistic. You like taking a leadership role and you are good at mastering new skills and teaching others. You like freedom and flexibility because this allows you to have the control to adjust your routine. When you connect passionately to a sport, your inner champion emerges.

FIT Reinforcers for the Spirited Planner: Nothing is more motivating to you than measurable results — results you can feel both physically and emotionally on your quest to optimal health and fitness.

Your love of nature makes the outdoors a great place to do some of your best thinking. List in your FIT Journal your goals and how you are doing. Add notes to this journal on what you learn about yourself and others on your fitness journey. This is a good way to feed your mind. It will provide you with new information as you master your workouts. Your FIT Journal can become a great resource for you to share your experiences with others who may be looking for pointers on how to stay motivated in their fitness.

FIT Detractors for the Spirited Planner: Be sure to balance your personal fitness time with the responsibilities you tend to take on. It is important for you to stay connected with your inner self and stay consistent in your exercise routine. Your natural love of connecting with people is a positive strength. Just be sure to devote equal time to yourself. These private moments will prove to be rejuvenating: a good way to stay systematic and structured in your fitness plan.

FIT Activities for the Spirited Planner: badminton, canoeing, cross-country skiing, golf, hiking, indoor cycling class, judo, mountain biking, nature walks, rock climbing, running with a partner, tai chi, tennis, yoga.

COMPETITIVE PERFORMER

If you scored **32–40** points you are a *Competitive Performer*, the play-to-win type.

You have a strong achievement orientation. As a competitive performer you strive hard to reach a goal. You tend to be interested in personal achievement and likely play to win when you take on a challenge.

Your practical style represents an independent, determined type. You are ambitious and persistent to be the best you can be, and you have a strong will to always cross the finish line.

You are the type who takes training seriously. The thought of performing better than the average keeps your internal flame burning. You train best when you have something to work toward. A competitive goal keeps you focused and motivated.

FIT Reinforcers for the Competitive Performer: Registering for an upcoming sporting event in your community will certainly keep your competitive spirit energized. The sign-up process and planning your training program for the event will get your adrenaline flowing. Your love of self-improvement can be nurtured by picking up an information-filled training book. Begin to track your training days in your Weekly FIT Training Log, adding a few notes about how you are feeling, the food you have been eating, and what you have learned as you train for the event. Keep motivated, evaluating your progress at the end of a week. Look for ways to optimize your program.

FIT Detractors for the Competitive Performer: You thrive in environments that challenge you. The driver within you needs to keep moving, so be sure to keep those competitive goals always in the forefront. Seek environments that nurture self-improvement. Also be cognizant of your need for recovery periods and don't overdo your training. Too much of a good thing can lead to injury and burnout. Nurture your inner competitive performer and reward yourself for your hard work.

FIT Activities for the Competitive Performer: dragon boat team racing, golf, indoor cycling classes, karate, outdoor cycling with a road bike group, running events, specialized dance classes, such as ballroom, salsa, tango, swimming, taekwondo, tennis, triathlons, weight training, yoga.

SELF-DIRECTED SOLOIST	CREATIVE DESIGNER
Compatible FIT Activities	**Compatible FIT Activities**
gardening, home training videos, horseback riding, ice-skating, indoor/outdoor cycling, in-line skating, jogging, mini-trampoline, swimming, walking, weight training, and yoga.	high/low impact aerobic classes, basketball, baseball, curling, folk dancing, frisbee, indoor/outdoor cycling, Pilates, running (with a partner or group), square dancing, tai chi, volleyball, weight training, in a muscle works class, water aerobics, yoga.
SPIRITED PLANNER	COMPETITIVE PERFORMER
Compatible FIT Activities	**Compatible FIT Activities**
badminton, canoeing, skiing, golf, hiking, indoor cycling class, mountain biking, nature walks, rock climbing, running with a partner, tai chi, tennis, yoga.	dragon boat team racing, golf, indoor cycling classes, karate, outdoor cycling with a road bike group, running events, specialized dance classes, such as ballroom, salsa, tango, swimming, taekwondo, tennis, triathlons, weight training, yoga.

Note: Review your FIT Motivational Style™ activities. Experiment by sampling activities that fit your own style as well as ones from the style closest to your score. Be curious and confident as you try out your FIT possibilities. Get ready to develop and nurture a stronger connection with your fitness.

YOUR IDEAL FIT ENVIRONMENT IS ...

VISUALIZE YOUR STYLE AND SUPPORTING ACTIVITIES

You have defined your FIT Motivational Style™ and have gained knowledge from the information you have read. Your left brain has been actively processing material in a logical, sequential manner and evaluating the steps you need to take in order to get moving.

By following the Guided Visualization Exercise below, you will turn on your right brain controls and begin to embark on integrating the information you have learned. The exercise requires you to use all of your senses — sight, taste, touch, smell, and hearing — including muscular sensations. You will create an experience that will guide you to a place where you can actually begin to develop a relationship with your FIT Motivational Style™. Your sense of awareness will be heightened and your confidence in your ability will expand.

This type of exercise is usually done with eyes closed, so if possible record yourself reading the script. Be sure to read it slowly and quietly, with no distracting sounds in the background. If you are not able to tape the script, then let us send you one. Just e-mail us at powersourceforwomen@gmail.com and place in the heading "Request for guided visualization." Tell us the format you prefer. We can send you a CD (please include your mailing address) or we can e-mail you an MP3 for downloading.

TAKE OUR 10-MINUTE
GUIDED VISUALIZATION EXERCISE

Before you get comfortable, select an activity from your FIT Motivational Style list. Keep that activity in the back of your mind; you will be revisiting it later in your visualization.

Now take a moment to settle down and get into a comfortable, upright position. Be sure to sit in a chair that supports good posture. Do not sit in one that allows you to slouch. We want you to be actively visualizing and not falling asleep.

Let's begin.

THE FOLLOWING IS TO BE READ SLOWLY. PAUSE APPROXIMATELY FIVE SECONDS AFTER EACH LINE. THIS EXERCISE WILL TAKE YOU LESS THAN 10 MINUTES TO COMPLETE.

Notice at this moment how you are feeling.

How are you doing at this very moment?

Pay attention to your thoughts.

What are you thinking?

How does your body feel?

Now begin slowly scanning your body with your mind.

Start by focusing your mind on scanning your feet.

Notice the sensation of your toes … the bottoms of your feet … your ankles … legs … hips …

Pay attention to your body and how it feels.

Notice how your lower back feels ... stomach ... chest ... your shoulders ...

Begin to move slowly down your arms and feel your wrist ... your palms ... each finger, starting with your thumb ...

Notice your neck ... head ... jaw ... face ...

Notice your mouth ... your nose ... your eyes ... and fore-head ...

Release any tension you feel in your forehead; feel the sen-sations of your scalp.

Begin to scan your body and notice any tension that you hold.

Where does your body feel the most relaxed?

Begin to feel a lightness in your body, as it relaxes naturally from sitting quietly and comfortably ... with no distractions.

Allow your body to continue to relax ... do not force your body ... just allow the relaxation to happen naturally.

You have been trying to connect with a more relaxed state for the last few moments. Let's take a step back now, men-tally, to relax.

Breathe in, slowly and deeply through your nose ... and breathe out slowly through your mouth. Create a circle or an "O" with your lips as if you were going to whistle to control and extend your rate of expiration.

In ... and out ...

In ... and out ...

In … and out …

Just relax for a moment and notice your breathing. You should be feeling a sense of calmness.

Now visualize how you see your body at this moment.

How do you feel about the image you see?

In your mind, begin to visualize how you would like to see your body.

Begin to sense how you feel in that new image.

Feel the energy you have.

Notice your mood lifting.

Keep that image in your mind until it is clear.

Begin to connect with your new image.

Holding that new image … breathe in, slowly and deeply, through your nose … and breathe out slowly through your mouth shaped like an "O."

Repeat …

Breathe in … and out …

Breathe in … and out …

Breathe in … and out …

Continue to hold your new image, while you begin to feel a renewed energy throughout your body.

Now begin to see yourself actively participating in the type of activity you selected as best suited to your FIT Motivational Style™.

See yourself enjoying the connection you are developing with the activity you have chosen.

Begin to feel how much more energized you are becoming as you connect further with your activity … with your body.

Notice what is around you as you participate in the physical activity you are enjoying.

Notice the scent of the environment.

Notice the colors in the environment.

Now … see the glow on your cheeks and notice the fun you are having.

Holding that image … breathe in, slowly and deeply through your nose … and breathe out slowly through your mouth shaped like an "O."

Repeat …

Breathe in … and out …

Breathe in … and out …

Breathe in … and out …

Now slowly begin to roll your shoulders back, five times.

Now slowly roll your shoulders forward, five times.

Sit quietly for one minute; gently smile as you think about your new image.

Think about the new relationship you are building with your fitness.

Now slowly begin to open your eyes.

JOURNALING WITH LESLEY SHORE

"Know your value. Confidence breeds success. Act like the person
you want to become, and people will start seeing you as that person."
–Michael Masterton

My FIT Motivational Style™ is Self-Directed Soloist with a touch of Creative Designer.

I think it would be more accurate to say that I'm a Self-Directed Soloist who harbors dreams of becoming a Creative Designer. I'm not there yet because I don't have the confidence in my body to join a real class. Warming up with the 90-year-olds in my condo fitness class on Thursday mornings is just right for me right now. Audrey, the teacher, tells me I can "ramp it up a little," but I'm content just to be able to do the exercises she models without wimping out.

One day, when my body feels stronger because I've stuck to my routine faithfully for a couple of months, I'll venture a toe in the water of a yoga class near my house. It seems important for me, at this point, not to have to venture too far from home to get my exercise — not to have to move too far out of my comfort zone.

What is absolutely certain is that I need the freedom to move at my own pace with this. Years of feeling intimidated in organized gym classes at school have taken their toll. I need to respect that. Slow and steady — like the tortoise. I'll get there.

START JOURNALING

Set your timer for 20 minutes for writing in your FIT Journal. What is your comfort zone when it comes to exercising? Write your thoughts about when it is right for you to stay in that zone and when it might be right for you to get out of it.

Power Source Tool #7

Create Your Own
FIT Action Plan

"The way to get started is to quit talking and begin doing."

–WALT DISNEY

Unrealistic fitness plans can be a recipe for failure, quickly turning your optimism and positive vision into a sea of doubt and despair. Make sure your plan includes time for the ups and downs of life and makes allowances for vacations, birthday parties, and other breaks.

The key is to base your fitness program on your motivational style, which you determined in the previous chapter.

Susan's Story

My FIT Motivational Style™ is Creative Designer, which perfectly describes my relationship with fitness: high energy with lots of body movement and variety in my fitness routines, as well as some quiet workouts.

I like the structure of classes, as well as the camaraderie. I have taken aerobics, step, and weights classes for over 20 years.

What has changed is that I have expanded my fitness schedule from three days a week to six days a week.

Since variety is very important to me, I have set up my schedule to do three strength-training and core-conditioning classes a week, as well as one spinning class, one morning of outdoor walking/jogging with my friend Pat, and, most recently, 60 minutes of walking/jogging on Saturday mornings on my own. I try to stretch after each workout, but often forget.

So far I have not been able to commit to yoga classes. Although I join a yoga class every once in a while, I get frustrated by my lack of flexibility, lose interest, and quickly give up. I envy people who do yoga. I have made it one of my future fitness goals.

Theresa's Story

My FIT Motivational Style™ is Spirited Planner, with a touch of the Competitive Performer style.

My love of running has developed as a result of the support and camaraderie that has been my source of inspiration from the beginning of my marathoning to my training today as I challenge myself with my 20th marathon. The friends I have gained through running are the reason I am where I am today. I enjoy the social component — it adds a human connectedness that makes my experience so much richer.

Teaching my Cycle Fit classes also provides me with the opportunity to be creative with music, moves, and physical demands. I have a great class of people at 6:15 a.m. on Tuesdays and 9:30 a.m. on Fridays. The chance to inspire and motivate the participants through my class has a positive effect on my mood as well as on my own fitness. The social component again proves to be an uplifting source of power. I enjoy sharing my fitness experience with them.

SEVEN STRATEGIES FOR CREATING YOUR OWN FIT ACTION PLAN

#1. Understand the key components of fitness
- Include four types of fitness in your FIT Action Plan: endurance, strength, balance, and flexibility.
- Start getting into shape with three one-hour exercise sessions per week. Combine aerobic exercise, strength training, and balance and flexibility exercises.
- Rotate different activities — such as walking, hiking, running, rowing, swimming, and cycling — to keep you moving while you condition various muscle groups. You could combine belly dance with yoga or jogging with weights to keep you from getting bored and make your fitness routine more effective.

#2. Be realistic about your current level of fitness before you create a plan
    Level 1: Beginning a fitness program
    Level 2: Returning to a fitness program
    Level 3: Expanding your fitness program

#3. Listen to your body
- Notice any aches, pains, or injuries when you start your workout. Analyze your energy level.
- Use your warm-up to become aware of your negative thoughts. If you find yourself thinking, "I'm so tired!" replace the thought with a positive inner dialogue.
- Use your cool-down to take inventory. Assess what you liked and what didn't work. What would you keep or change in your workout plan?

- Evaluate the impact on your body. You may feel some soreness and breathlessness after a workout, but you should not feel dizzy, nauseous, or short of breath. If you have these signals, stop exercising and check your fitness plan with your doctor.
- After each workout, track your progress, in writing, in your Weekly FIT Training Log.

#4. Set up your own home gym and a traveling gym

Following are seven suggestions for inexpensive (or free) types of equipment ideal for a home gym or to pack for traveling. You can often find barely used fitness items such as exercise DVDs, workout clothes, home gym equipment, and more at yard sales, garage sales, or online community boards. ❄

When you go on vacation, check out the fitness facilities where you'll be staying and bring along your exercise clothes and equipment, including resistance bands, a bathing suit, shorts, t-shirts, and workout shoes.

1. **Resistance bands**

Stretchy and fun, these elastic bands do the work of weights for strength-training exercises and pack easily in a purse or pocket. They come in a number of strengths and colors and can be used for several body areas. Choose a light band if you are starting to exercise; then move to heavier bands.

2. **Jumping rope**

Just five or 10 minutes of jumping (indoors or outdoors) will boost your activity level and burn calories.

3. **Exercise mat**

A mat is more comfortable and safer for exercise than a carpet, shiny surface, or wooden floor.

4. Free weights

Keep a set of hand weights or dumbbells by your computer or television set and use these during commercials or throughout the day. Purchase a range of weights for different exercises.

You can also use homemade weights for a Green FIT program. Try filling a plastic milk jug with water or sand, or fill a sock with dried beans and tie the end. 🌟

5. Exercise balls

Exercise balls are sized for your height. Most come with their own pump for easy inflation. They are great for traveling and for strengthening various muscle groups. You can sit on the ball in front of the computer; you'll get a workout just from balancing on it. The ball will improve the stability of your joints and promote balance and core conditioning.

6. Pedometer or step counter

Wear a pedometer and you'll become more aware of how much (or little) you're moving every day. The American Heart Association and other experts suggest ten thousand steps per day. Increase to fifteen thousand steps a day for additional benefits.

7. Step-stool

A low, solid step-stool can be used as a piece of equipment for step training, which has a similar effect to climbing stairs.

#5. Our Functional FIT Workout Plan — 20 to 30 minutes to a stronger, healthier you

Functional fitness has been getting a lot of attention in recent years since it prepares people for handling real-life movements and situations. For example, just bending down to pick something up can be a challenge for many people.

You can begin to build your level of functional fitness with seven simple exercises. Follow our Functional FIT Workout Plan below two or three times per week. You will find you are targeting the four key components of fitness: you are gaining flexibility and strength while also improving your balance and physical endurance.

OUR FUNCTIONAL FIT WORKOUT PLAN: SEVEN EXERCISES TO STRENGTHEN YOUR BODY

If you are new to Functional Fitness, start out slowly and spend about 20 minutes completing the exercises. As you get stronger, you will be able to extend your Functional Fitness Workout Plan to 30 minutes or more.

The Warm-up

1. Sit up with your back straight and your shoulders back. Your buttocks should touch the back of your chair.
2. Allow your arms to hang gently next to you.
3. Begin to slowly roll your shoulders in backward circles ten times.
4. Roll your shoulders in forward circles ten times (pay attention to your seated position: do not slouch).
5. Roll your neck slowly to the right making circles five times.
6. Roll your neck slowly to the left making circles five times.
7. Take a deep breath in through your nose, slowly expanding your belly as it fills with air. Be sure to

keep your shoulders down and relaxed as you breathe in. Now slowly exhale through your nose or through your mouth creating a cirlce or an "O" with your lips as if you were going to whistle. This helps you control your rate of expiration. Repeat three times.

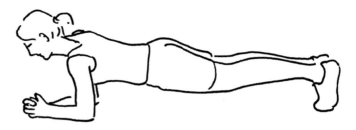

1. Core Strengthener

1. Lying face down on a mat, place your elbows and forearms underneath your chest.
2. Slowly lift yourself up to form a bridge using your toes and forearms.
3. Your back should be flat and your hips should not be sagging.
4. Begin to focus on tightening your abs while you hold this position. Hold this position to the count of 10 and then slowly lower your body and return to your start position.
5. Do this three times and, as your core gets stronger, hold the count longer.
6. To get the most out of this exercise, pull your belly button toward your spine.

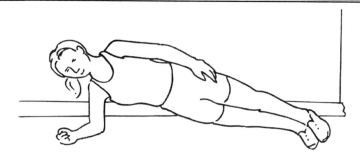

2. Side Plank Balancer

1. Lie on a mat, starting with this position on your right side.
2. Begin this exercise on your forearm. Lift yourself up to form a plank with your right arm, while keeping your elbow to the mat.
3. Hold to the count of five, slowly increasing to 10 and then 15 as you get stronger. Try to complete three sets.
4. Now move to your left side and repeat.
5. As you get stronger, begin to use a straight arm instead of the forearm to lift you up. Begin by starting on your side, resting on your hand.

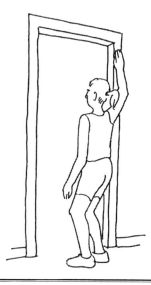

3. Shoulder Flexibility

1. In your home or office, stand in front of a door with a doorframe. Raise your hand on the side you want to stretch as high as you can. Now grasp the doorframe with the same hand.
2. Keeping your arm straight, lower your body by bending your knees. When you begin to feel the stretch in your shoulder, hold this stretch for the count

of five and then return to your start position. Repeat three times.

3. Be sure to keep your back straight. To maximize this stretch over time, try bending your knees slightly lower or raising your arm higher when you begin the exercise.

4. Work up to holding the stretch for 30 to 60 seconds.

4. Arm Strengthener

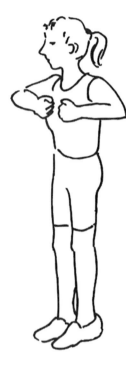

1. Stand with your arms folded inwards (elbows should be positioned out and hands pulled into chest), fists tucked close to the chest, elbows parallel to the floor.

2. Raise arms slowly upwards (not above the shoulders) and then backwards. Keep your fists tucked inwards as you perform this movement. Apply pressure as much as possible on the biceps and triceps. Hold to the count of five.

3. Return to your starting position and perform three repetitions.

4. As your arms get stronger, extend your hold count to 10, then 15 seconds.

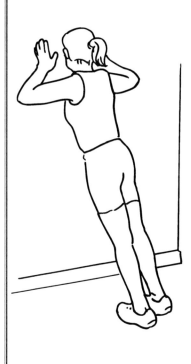

5. Wall Push-up

1. Stand facing a wall and extend your arms out in front of you.
2. Now lean forward slightly toward the wall and place your palms against the surface.
3. Take a deep breath in and slowly begin to exhale as you start to bend your elbows until your nose nearly touches the wall.
4. Slowly return to your start position and repeat. Do three sets of 10 to start and then increase the number of repetitions as your strength increases.

6. Extending Your Reach

1. Place a coin on the floor and take three steps back.
2. Slowly walk toward the coin.
3. Stop and lunge or squat down to pick up the coin and return to your standing position.
4. Re-place the coin on the floor and walk three steps away from the coin; turn to face it and repeat.
5. Do three repetitions and increase as your balance and coordination improve.

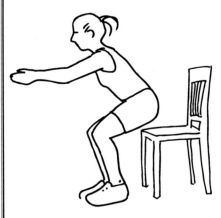

7. Leg Strengthener

1. Place a chair directly behind you and stand in front of it with your feet about hip- or shoulder-width apart.
2. Tighten your abs, holding them in; begin to bend your knees slowly into a squat toward the chair.
3. As you sit on the chair, be sure to keep your knees behind your toes.
4. Contract your glutes and hamstrings to lift you up out of your chair; then begin to extend your legs.
5. Extend your legs until you return to your standing position.
6. Do this exercise in reps of five to begin with and do one to three sets. As you get stronger, you can increase the number of repetitions per set and how often you do them.
7. To get even stronger, squat down until you are just above the chair — but not sitting down. Be sure to keep your knees in line with your toes.

#6. Make changes to your Functional FIT Workout Plan as you continue to work out.

- Regular self-monitoring of your exercises may be the single most important thing you can do to stay on track. Use a calendar or an electronic scheduling device to log your achievements.
- Recognize and acknowledge the things that don't work in your plan and be willing to change them.

#7. Create a Weekly FIT Training Log

- Create a Weekly FIT Training Log. Include the kinds of activities you will do, why you want to do them, and when and where you will exercise. This can help you to track where you have been and where you are going.
- Spend a few minutes each morning thinking or writing about what you want to accomplish that day and how you'll do it. Use Lesley Shore's suggestions for journaling at the end of each chapter of this book to track your thoughts and feelings. Releasing negative feelings and focusing on gratitude will lift your mood.
- Remind yourself of your goals and take some time to appreciate how far you've come in reaching them.
- Review your personal assessment six weeks after you start your program and then every three to six months. You may need to increase the amount of time you exercise, or you may be surprised to find you are doing the right amount of exercise to meet your fitness goals.

CREATE YOUR WEEKLY FIT TRAINING LOG

Use the following sample to set up your own log.

MY WEEKLY FIT TRAINING LOG

WEEK OF

My fitness goal for the week is _____

Declaration Statement
I declare that

What are my needs in order to achieve my goal for the week? For example, one hour for me between 6 a.m. and 7 a.m. (be specific).

My Partners:
My training schedule (include times):
Sunday   _____
Monday   _____
Tuesday   _____
Wednesday _____
Thursday   _____
Friday   _____
Saturday _____

My body log (aches and pains):

My food log:

My mood log:
What was my overall attitude and mood this week?

What were my challenges?

How can I improve my training approach for next week?

GETTING STARTED WITH DORINA VENDRAMIN

I will soon be approaching 45 years of age, and it seems life is passing me by. I feel as if I let myself go in the past 10 years or so. I have been putting everyone else's needs in front of my own so as to not feel selfish, yet I find myself living in guilt for not being there more for everyone.

The truth is I am cheating the number one person out of time and that someone is me.

About a year and a half ago my family doctor Claudia Petrescu referred me to see a psychiatrist specializing in weight loss, Dr. Barry Simon. Since meeting Dr. Simon and rejoining Weight Watchers, I have lost 40 pounds. Recently I heard Susan Sommers was writing a book with Theresa Dugwell about women over 45 who use exercise as their way of managing the stress in their lives. So I decided to ask Susan if she would mind taking on a "student in training" as a makeover person.

The time has come in my life to take another step toward getting back into the groove of living versus watching it go by.

Every day I must make a decision whether to revert to my old habits or move forward. In all honesty I have had many setbacks as I'm sure many of you have. What I work on most is trying not to beat up on myself for straying and focusing on getting back on track.

I am grateful to have met the women in this book and for their caring enough to want to help me be the best I can be. I suppose what drives me most is the doing this for myself now, while others are supporting me. I don't want to regret not trying to get healthy and fit while I had such a good cheerleading team behind me.

SAMPLES FROM DORINA VENDRAMIN'S WEEKLY FIT TRAINING LOG

My FIT Weekly Log

WEEK OF _March_ **1**st - _March **7**th_

My Fitness Goal For The Week is _Look in front of mirror, try to look back._

---- Declaration Statement ----

I declare that _____

_____

Promise to Self

I promise to _____

What are my needs in order to achieve my goal for the week?
ie. One Hour for me between 6am – 7am [be specific about your needs]

Call Sandra re: Christine

_____

Training Schedule

Sunday _____
Monday _____
Tuesday _Walk @ lunch 30 minutes_   Count
Wednesday _stairs x Walked @ lunch 30 minutes_   many
Thursday _Walk @ lunch 30 minutes._
Friday _stairs_
Saturday _weekend walk or Sunday_

Reflections and Comments (What was my overall attitude and mood this week? What were my challenges? How can I improve my training approach for next week?)

_____
_____
_____
_____

Your "FIT" Weekly Log

WEEK OF _Mar 8 – Mar 14_

My Fitness Goal For The Week is _____

Declaration Statement

I declare that _track food, 4 min walk with walk/day. 2 waters_
2 throughout day.

Promise to Self

I promise to _drink 4 – 8oz glasses of water_
per day 2 before or 2 after

What are my needs in order to achieve my goal for the week?
ie. One Hour for me between 6am – 7am [be specific about your needs]

Try to keep motivating myself through
motivating others

Training Schedule

Sunday _____
Monday _30 minute walk_
Tuesday _luncheon — walked show_
Wednesday _30 minute walk_
Thursday _30 minute walk_
Friday _30 minute walk_
Saturday _____

Reflections and Comments (What was my overall attitude and mood this week? What were my challenges? How can I improve my training approach for next week?)

Little down due to Menstral & 2 lb gain
_at WW._
Didn't get a weekend walk in!

Journalling — who's been helping me along
the way ⊙WW

Grateful for having met motivational women
this past Sunday PowerWomen

Your "FIT" Weekly Log

WEEK OF _Mar 15 – Mar 21_

My Fitness Goal For The Week is _____

Declaration Statement

I declare that _____

Promise to Self

I promise to _____

What are my needs in order to achieve my goal for the week?
ie. One Hour for me between 6am – 7am [be specific about your needs]

Less TV, more me time in the evening
Give Myself

Training Schedule

Sunday _Picture @ Y, Mom's_   Down
Monday _____   3 lbs @
Tuesday _TAXES_   WW
Wednesday _Walk 30 minutes_   trying to get
Thursday _Walk 30 minutes._   back to where
Friday _Walk 30 minutes._   I first started
Saturday _No activity - cleaned closet_ going again

Reflections and Comments (What was my overall attitude and mood this week? What were my challenges? How can I improve my training approach for next week?)

★ Food was challenging
Activity at lunch feels do able
Weekends seem to be more to get
things done, help others, must take/make
time for me.
Guilt around not being there for others, but
also for not being there for myself.

Drinking More Water

My FIT Weekly Log

WEEK OF _Mar 22 - 28_

My Fitness Goal For The Week is _to attempt a weekend activity_

Declaration Statement

I declare that _I will put myself first this coming_
weekend and do an activity to help me
get to my fitness goals!

Promise to Self

I promise to _DO MY BEST, take time for me_
X Research _- learn to walk_
X _look for runners_

What are my needs in order to achieve my goal for the week?
ie. One Hour for me between 6am – 7am [be specific about your needs]

X _spend Tuesday evenings as night for me._
Call Theresa for weekly check in, work on
X _Vision Board / journal / me time!_
X _Call Christine 416 253 5177_

Training Schedule

Sunday _____
Monday _____
✓ Tuesday _Walk 30 minutes_
✓ Wednesday _Walk 30 minutes_ X _Ewen Rd Plant Visit/Interview_
X Thursday _Walk 30 minutes - ? work from home /interview_
X Friday _Walk 30 minutes - ? work from home /interview_
✓ Saturday _Walk / garden / other 30-60 minutes or more_

Reflections and Comments (What was my overall attitude and mood this
week? What were my challenges? How can I improve my training approach
for next week?)

_____
_____
_____
_____
_____
_____

My FIT Weekly Log

WEEK OF _Mar 29 - april 4th_

My Fitness Goal For The Week is _going to be less walking during_
the day due to other
Declaration Statement _appointments_

I declare that _._
_____
_____

Promise to Self

I promise to _try to stop feeling guilt around_
not staying on track!

What are my needs in order to achieve my goal for the week?
ie. One Hour for me between 6am – 7am [be specific about your needs]

_____
_____
_____

Training Schedule

Sunday _Easter -_
Monday _Doctors for Physical_
Tuesday _Hockey Game - Overate / interview_
✓ Wednesday _cleaning evening for party._
Thursday _Dinner Party - Not ate drunk._
✓ Friday _Good Friday Garden - 3+ hours_
✓ Saturday _Garden - 3+ hours washed car._

Reflections and Comments (What was my overall attitude and mood this
week? What were my challenges? How can I improve my training approach
for next week?)

Felt very out of shape and sore after
gardening which made me realize I
must get some control back again
so yardwork doesn't hurt
Did not go to Weight Watchers and
also cancelled Dr. Simon

JOURNALING WITH LESLEY SHORE

"Don't fear change, embrace it." –Goethe

Remember the good old days when running on the spot was considered exercise? Guess what? It still is. Now I've bought the equipment: the jump rope, the resistance bands, the gym mat, the weighted balls, and the exercise videos where all those gorgeous girls and women in their bright and sassy gym clothes parade their nearly perfect bodies before me.

I like the weighted ball workout the best. But I can be humbled by all this enthusiasm, even intimidated. There are times when I avoid these smiling, happy creatures.

But I don't mind running back and forth along the upstairs hallway for ten minutes. I know it makes a better start to my day if I take the time to do it. I carry heavy but balanced loads home from the local grocery store a few times a week instead of taking the car. And every day I whip up and down the two sets of stairs in my townhouse more times than I can count. The woman who lived here before me was 89 and was still climbing the stairs. "They're my exercise," she used to say.

Hats off to Dorina Vendramin for having the discipline to keep a FIT Training Log.

Keeping one would surely help me to keep on track. Am I disciplined enough to do it for one week and see what a difference it might make in making me accountable to a routine? Are you? One week doesn't seem too much to ask of ourselves.

PART 3

Emotional Fitness: Change Your Life

Power Source Tool #8

Recognize Challenges, Persevere, and Refocus on Your Fitness Goals

"It's okay to have doubts;
just don't feed and entertain them."

–JOHN IRVING

We are two-thirds of the way along on our journey together. Parts 1 and 2 of this book dealt with mental and physical fitness. Let's turn now, in this third and final part, to emotional fitness. We have placed this discussion last because, as you will see, emotional fitness is closely tied to physical fitness.

If you're like most of us, you resist change. Stress, excitement, doubt, and fear are emotions you may feel when you start — and as you're sustaining — a fitness program.

You don't always know what fitness obstacles or setbacks are coming or even recognize them when they occur.

Sometimes they are money related (you can't afford to continue at a gym), or family related (care-giving responsibilities, family illness, or the death of a loved one), or time related (too busy with work or family responsibilities).

Sometimes they involve physical problems, such as injury and various illnesses.

For some people the obstacles are emotional, such as depression, hormone imbalances, sleep apnea, food allergies, unhealthy relationships, perfectionism, or addiction.

In addition, because you may not see changes right away — in your body shape or on the scale — you may be afraid your fitness program is not working. This can confirm your previous doubts and fears about never being able to get fit.

Don't listen to your negative inner voice, the one that doesn't want discomfort or inconvenience. It will deplete the power source within you. View setbacks as learning experiences: assess your feelings, understand the problems and obstacles, and find different ways to persevere and reconnect.

The feeling that comes from believing that you're enhancing your life will make it easier for you to embrace the changes. Concentrate on the whole experience, both the good and the bad. Stay focused on the solution, not on the problem.

Susan's Story

My biggest physical obstacle to completing two marathons was lower back pain. My biggest mental obstacle was fear — that I would not be able to keep moving for over seven hours to complete the races. I knew that five hours of walking and jogging during my training was about all I could muster. It would therefore take more of a mental effort than a physical one for me to keep moving beyond that point.

It was always at this juncture that I had to find ways to motivate myself to finish. Sometimes it helped if I started to talk to someone nearby — that took my mind off how much time I had left. Then I would go back on my own.

For my second marathon, in 2007, the obstacles were overwhelming. By the time I had completed the race, the roads had reopened, the sun was blazing, the toilets were packed away, and the bottles of water were gone. There was no finish line, no medal, and no cheering crowds. The organizers had already packed up and left, and the Scotiabank Waterfront Marathon website listed me as "did not finish."

The one person waiting for me to come in was my daughter, Danielle. In fact, it was sheer determination, self-affirmation, and singing that got me through both marathons — and the help of my husband Peter and my friend Pat, who were by my side when I crossed the finish line.

Theresa's Story

Because I finish work late many nights, it can be difficult for me to get to the gym early enough the next day to run with the running group. In order to make this possible, I set everything out the night before. That way I can jump out of bed when the alarm goes off, quickly put on my workout clothes, grab my cup of chai, and head out the door with my gym bag ready to go.

It's critical for me to keep up the momentum from the time I get out of bed until the moment I hit the gym. Once I arrive, the energy from the environment activates my mind and motivates me to get my body moving.

SEVEN STRATEGIES FOR RECOGNIZING CHALLENGES, PERSEVERING, AND REFOCUSING ON YOUR FITNESS GOALS

#1. *Acknowledge and accept your challenges*
- When you hit the inevitable stumbling blocks and obstacles, keep going — even when you feel sluggish or don't see the benefits of exercise. There will be times when you'll just get by and other times when you'll sail through. Persistence is the key.

- Find the incentives you need to motivate you. Realize that you are tougher on yourself than you are on others. Take a look back and see how you got to where you are today. Chances are, you'll see a path of persistence, perseverance, and progress. Look for continuous improvement over time.
- Talk to your doctor, accountability team, family, or friends about your desire to get back on track.

#2. Center yourself and slow down your thoughts
- Be fully present in your life.
- First thing in the morning, pause and bless the day. Take a few deep breaths. Add breaks throughout your day to reconnect with your spiritual essence and to express gratitude. Set aside time for yourself.

#3. Incorporate stress-reduction tools into your daily life and into your fitness routine
Always be present in your fitness class or workout. Don't let your mind wander. Here are some strategies and tools that will help you:

Mindfulness and meditation
The more you build silent moments into your life, the more you'll be able to experience a quiet state of mind anywhere, even in the midst of the chaos of life.
- Set aside quiet time for yourself each day and meditate. Find a place inside yourself where you can be totally peaceful in order to enhance your total health.
- Take a silent lunch: no cell phones, text messaging, or reading.

- Linger at a park bench.
- Stop and smell the roses.

Inspirational quotes and strong statements
Strong statements increase your belief, confidence, and motivation. Think about these on a daily basis and analyze what they mean to you.
- Create desktop wallpaper with quotes and sayings you love and post quotes on your bathroom mirror or your wall. They will give you the visual inspiration to overcome obstacles and stay motivated.
- Listen to relaxation CDs, such as Tibetan chants and Buddhist meditations.

#4. Create a vision board
We asked Monika Klein, one of our Power Source Women, to define and describe the benefits of Vision Boards. She is the President of Coaching for Health, LLC, a California-based company devoted to health and wellness, and she works with vision boards in her private practice.

I have been using Vision Boards as a personal development tool for myself as well as for my clients for years. It is a powerful technique that can help clarify your goals, priorities, and dreams and can perhaps reveal a strategy for how to accomplish them. Vision Boards are now being used increasingly in corporate and business environments for team building and leadership development as well. This magical tool can help you engage your imagination.

By using images and words found in magazines you create a collage-like picture filled with things that appeal to you. You can gain better insight as to what kind of future

*you'd like to have and what's important to you. These
images can often inspire certain feelings, giving you the
essence of what you want to create. For example, you may
want more quiet time so you pick a picture of a beach scene,
or you want more freedom so you pick a picture of a plane
or an eagle in flight. You can choose whatever you like.
What's important is that it means something to you.*

*When putting your Vision Board together, try not
analyze or think too much about the image you've chosen.
Don't try to be perfect. Just allow your right brain — your
creative and imaginative side — free rein. By doing this you
are letting your playful and uncensored self tell you not only
your most obvious wishes in visual form but also some inner
yearnings you didn't know you had.*

*I enjoy incorporating Vision Boards into my work. When
helping my clients with their health and wellness, I often
recommend this fun and powerful tool to help them visualize
what they want. Since I often work with individuals wanting
to lose weight, I use the Vision Board process to help them
envision their future self — how they'd like to look. Even
after losing weight, this tool assists them in identifying with a
new leaner self-image versus an older, outdated one that is no
longer applicable to their new reality.*

*This process can often provide an authentic solution
to a person's problem even when that person is stuck. The
psychological-healing benefit of the Vision Board process is
immense. It takes a person on an inner journey and gives
them a creative roadmap.*

#5. Develop your own mantra
We asked Power Source Women to describe their own "self-
talk" — the mantras that keep them focused and get them

---

through each workout, week, and race. Pick the ones that will work for you.

- One more rep.
- 10 more minutes on the cardio machine.
- Stop looking at the time indicator.
- You've done five miles before. It wasn't hard.
- You're almost done.
- Spring is here.
- Come on, you've done great so far — just a bit more.
- Madonna.
- It will all be worth it in the end. It always is.
- If it's not getting harder — and it's not — then there's no reason I can't keep going.
- Bikini! Bikini! Bikini!
- I will look great in my clothes — and out of them.
- I started this, I can finish it.
- Did you get up this morning just to quit halfway through?
- You can do anything for one minute.
- What doesn't kill me can only make me stronger.
- Get sexy, get sexy, get sexy!
- What else do you have to do right now? You're here, you might as well finish.
- Running is a dance party, and it's easier at the end.
- Suck it up, buttercup.
- Float, float, float with every step.
- Demi Moore didn't quit in GI Jane.
- Just do it and get it over with. You'll feel so good afterwards.
- Better. Faster. Stronger.
- Pain is temporary but pride is forever.
- Come on, come on, just five more minutes.

- Man, who is that sexy girl running?
- My body is a temple.
- My legs are a powerhouse.
- You can do this. Your body can do this.

These women also said:

- I go through my play list until I get to "Stronger" by Kanye West. Apart from being incredibly motivational to me, making me feel like a lean mean exercise machine (ha ha), I always remember how Katie Holmes said listening to this song on repeat was what got her through running a marathon. That makes me think that my exercise program is nothing even close to a marathon and somehow that makes it all feel easier.
- The right music gets me through. JT and Madonna's song "Four Minutes" is *perfect* to help push me through the last four minutes of my cardio.
- Thinking about Madonna makes me realize that if she can do it at nearly 50, I can, too. Anyway, what would I be doing if I weren't exercising right now? Probably eating junk food and getting fat.
- There are two types of people in this world: those who say, "I can't!" and those who say, "I will never accept defeat."
- My imaginary coach always congratulates me after a good workout and adds, "Next time you'll do even better."
- When I start to feel fatigued or negative, I smile or imagine myself smiling. The act seems to really boost my mood and gives me the push when I give it a try.

> #### #6. *Stay connected with other people*
> An important external motivator is a connection with someone or something else: a doctor, a trainer, an exercise group, a nutrition expert, a friend or family member, or an online forum or blog. Welcome the support and encouragement of other people.
>
> #### #7. *Change your fitness program when you hit a plateau*
> Take a different approach. Try to modify your current program to change your experience and open up new possibilities. If you've been focusing on aerobic activity and not on strength training, switch your routine. Vary your meals and snacks. Stay focused on your goal and explore different ways to achieve it.
>
> Always have a backup plan. Be willing to change your plans if you find you're tired one day or you have to work late.

OUR POWER SOURCE EXPERT, RUTH KRONGOLD, SPEAKS

I deal with doubts and fears by doing something about them. I try to slow my thoughts down, assess how I am feeling, identify what the problems are, and develop some different options for my action plan. Imagination is my main resource in overcoming obstacles. Taking a walk or a swim, talking to a trusted ally, or just spending some time in a natural setting also helps.

Physical and emotional adaptations often assist me in overcoming obstacles. It takes work to create and maintain access to the things that bring meaning and pleasure into my life in spite of the inevitable changes that occur. As life progresses, I find it very useful to bring consciousness and intentionality to the choices I make about which life stories to keep, which to edit, and which to throw away. Making conscious choices gives me an active part in the unfolding of my own life story.

When doubts and fears overwhelm me, I seek assistance from friends, family, and professionals. A feeling of well-being, a connection with natural beauty and loved ones, being alive and able to appreciate what life has to offer in any moment, and being able to make a positive contribution — all of these things motivate me to work at being as healthy and fit as I can be.

OUR POWER SOURCE WOMEN SPEAK

We asked our Power Source Women to describe their challenges and how they overcome them. We asked them to fill us in on how they keep themselves motivated.

Audrey

I travel quite a bit and it is often difficult to fit fitness in. People say, "Oh, but you walk." I don't really think of walking as fitness so it's important that I do more than that. In places like India or China, that's more difficult. Ever since I started skipping in my boxing classes, the skipping rope has become my constant suitcase companion. I usually also pack a physio resistance strap and use it to practice my boxing technique and for upper body training. I always resolve to do sit-ups and push-ups, which would be nice, but I seldom get around to them.

There have been times in the last 20 years when my job forced me to exercise early in the morning and I was a regular at 6 a.m. classes; other times I was at the office by that time so I exercised at 7:30 or 8:30 p.m. I was lucky enough to belong to a club that had fitness classes at those times. Most people say they hate classes because their lives are too busy for them to commit to any particular time, but I haven't found that to be a problem.

I stay motivated because I'm too old to do things I don't love. So I stopped fooling myself that I would go on a treadmill or a stationary bike at a dingy hotel gym. Or use a universal gym weight machine. Instead, if possible, I take classes at a local gym. It's easier in North America or England, of course, but I've also taken step classes in a variety of languages: German, Italian, and French.

Edna

My challenge is to overcome my occasional doubts and fears that my health will fail. So far these have not become obstacles. I overcome them by *pushing* them to the back of my mind. I stay motivated because I am determined to accomplish something with my life.

Pat

Fitting everything into a busy schedule and staying motivated are my challenges. The buddy system is essential for me; so is knowing how to arrange my workouts so I feel rejuvenated. Exercise is always part of my day, not something I do only when it's convenient.

Phyllis

One of my biggest struggles has been getting myself out of bed in the morning to go to the gym. I have had challenges with my early-morning body and my feet ache, which sometimes makes getting up a challenge. But when I reflect on how good I will feel once I get there, something comes over me and suddenly I feel motivated to move my body, get out of bed, do some light stretches, and head for the gym.

RUTH KRONGOLD ON FITNESS
AS A MEDITATIVE PRACTICE

As both a meditative and fitness practice, swimming continues to give me a sense of myself as healthy and strong. This is energizing and highly motivating for me. It is also a lot of fun.

Long-distance fitness activities require a commitment of time and energy. The rewards show themselves slowly in two ways: an ongoing sense of physical and mental well-being and an increased resilience in the face of setbacks. These activities can be an effective antidote to depression and anxiety. They can facilitate the work of emotional and physical recovery.

When I do my morning swim, for example, I breathe evenly for about an hour and a half. While I may at times kick harder or try to push my cardio workout, breathing is the focus and center of my swim. Breath awareness is essential in the water to avoid drowning. This is a surprisingly difficult concept.

Being mindful of breath while swimming creates the opportunity for me to appreciate the present moment, attending to aches or pains that may occur, to thoughts and problems as they drift through consciousness, but always returning to the breath that sustains life. As T. S. Eliot writes in *Four Quartets*, "We shall not cease from exploration / And the end of all our exploring / Will be to arrive where we started / And know the place for the first time."

No matter how low I might feel physically or emotionally when I enter the water, I always feel better when I get out. Although it is not my intention to solve problems while I swim, giving myself this regular focused time without distractions allows my mind to rest and formulate otherwise inaccessible creative ideas.

Connection to the natural world is an important part of my life, and fitness helps to keep the possibility of that link vibrant. An indescribable feeling of awe and happiness comes over me when I turn to take a breath while swimming freestyle in a calm lake as the cool morning mist is rising and I find myself looking into the red eye of a loon. These moments are like magic. I feel included in something unique and beautiful.

The peace of evening paddles at sunset, walking, skiing, or snowshoeing through some of the most beautiful terrain on earth, whether alone or with loved ones — this peace would not be possible for me without a background of fitness.

OUR ROLE MODEL #4: GLORIA JACOBS

MY STORY

Seven years ago I embarked on a journey. I responded to an announcement at work that a dragon boat team was being formed — no experience necessary. My interest was twofold: I saw it as an unusual networking opportunity and as a chance to experience an unknown sport.

I was no novice to athletics. I had always worked out: free weights, weight machines, running, biking, aerobics, and dance. I knew next to nothing about dragon boating. I knew it was a team sport and that the activity was paddling. I had no idea that I would be walking into a completely new community of people who would introduce me to a whole new world of possibilities.

My introduction to the sport started off slowly and gently. The team met in the evening at a swimming pool. We each picked up a wooden paddle, sat down on a spot behind each other along the sides of the pool, and met our coach, Joe. By the end of the first season, I was seriously hooked.

During the second year, it quickly became obvious to me that, although paddling had started off as just one of my workout activities, I now was working out in order to paddle better.

I became intrigued with the idea of training to try out for a spot on the Canadian Masters team. I had an opportunity to paddle with some of the current members of the team and it felt good. I thought to myself, "I can do this. I belong in this boat."

Joe echoed my thoughts and said if I wanted it, he would take me there. And so I began a rigorous training schedule: three days a week with him and another three days a week on my own. As I became physically stronger than I ever dreamed I could, I began to think I could achieve everything I needed to. Physical strength translated into mental empowerment for me.

MY FITNESS PROGRAM

My attempt to move up in the paddling world had not gone unnoticed. I was invited to be a part of the Canadian National team in a new exhibition category — Grand Dragons — at the World Dragon Boat competition in Berlin in the summer of 2005. This would be my first international elite athletic experience and I was determined to be ready for it.

I had experienced the wonderful journey of physical empowerment and now was face to face with the reality of elite athletics. Sport competition at the world level is about winning. It's about grit and determination, the killer instinct, and never giving up. Coaches are there to win with a winning team. Each individual on a team is responsible to both themselves and their teammates to give 100 percent plus all the time. No one ever willingly admits weakness, or wants to be seen as a weak link. The purity of taking part takes a back seat to winning.

MY WAKE-UP CALL

In April 2007, after my annual mammogram, I was called back for some additional pictures. I have a strong history of breast cancer in my family and always had the nagging feeling it would not be if, but when, it would be my turn. My first questions for the doctors were also about paddling — when I could start again.

My doctors encouraged me to go forward. They didn't have any answers as to how much strength I would lose, or if I could recover in time, but they knew that striving to reach this goal and staying as active as I could be was very important for the health of my mind and body.

MY SOLUTION

I was adamant in trying, yet at the same time I had doubts. The first qualifying training camp weekend on the Gatineau River loomed ahead of me. Any activity, particularly athletics, is 80 percent mental. I wasn't sure I belonged there and had my worst time trials. I was devastated. I did not tell any teammates what I was facing.

By the end of May, I had a lumpectomy, luckily with no other involvement. I missed three weeks of training and told no one on the team why. Elite athletic competition is not a democracy. Although the women on my team would be sympathetic, I knew that inwardly they would be dismissing me. I would be seen as a weak link.

Training through recovery and radiation was not pleasant, but the alternative was not an option for me. Breast cancer would not define me: it was just something that happened. I persevered, kept my spot on the team, competed in Australia, and, together with the team, brought home a silver medal and a bronze medal.

TAKE GLORIA JACOBS'S INSPIRATIONAL QUIZ

Achieve It! As George Eliot said, "It's never too late to become the person you were meant to be."

Lesson 1
"Throw a pebble into a pond. It sends a shiver across the surface of the water. Ripples merge into one another and create new ones."
–Sogyal Rinpoche, *The Tibetan Book of Living and Dying*
Research your new opportunity
Do a risk analysis
Identify your fears

---

*Identify one thing you would like to do. It can be anything
— but just one thing:*

_____

Lesson 2
"My chief want in life is someone who shall make me do what
I can." – Ralph Waldo Emerson
Pay attention to people around you as potential role models, including the negative ones.
Establish a support network to help you achieve your goals.
*Name someone you know who could give you information
about what you would like to do:*

_____

Lesson 3
"The greatest human freedom is the freedom to choose one's attitude." – Viktor Frankl, Man's Search for Meaning
Practice positive thinking
Repeat positive affirmations
Acknowledge your feelings … now get on with the job.

Write down three negative thoughts about yourself:
1.

2.

3.

Write down three positive thoughts about yourself.
1.

2.

3.

Lesson 4

"This — the immediate, everyday and present experience — is IT, the entire, and ultimate point for the existence of a universe."
–Alan Watts, *This Is It: and Other Essays on Zen and Spiritual Experience*

Draw your design for living, incorporating balance between:

    Work and play

    Family and self

    Responsibility and desire

Name something that makes you truly happy:

_____

Lesson 5

"The Lance Armstrong Foundation's 'Live Strong' motto is about spreading hope and inspiration to the cancer community and adopting a positive attitude to face difficult circumstances — to live strong in the face of adversity. It's critical to remain positive, whether it's at work, racing a bike, or fighting an illness."
–Lance Armstrong

Listen to your body and work with it.

Transform a problem, even a big one, into a challenge.

View a setback as an opportunity for personal growth.

What is one step you could take today to move toward your goal?

_____

_____

JOURNALING WITH LESLEY SHORE

"As you go the way of life, you will come to a great chasm.
Jump. It is not as far as you think." –Native American saying

One of the benefits of keeping a journal is the perspective it gives you to look back and see your progress. Reading my earlier entries remind me both of how committed I was to make my own changes and how fearful at the same time. But that commitment was the fire in my belly. I was moving ahead, full speed ahead.

Then there were three weeks when I was laid up with the stomach flu, had to stick close to my toilet, and spent most of my time in bed. How would I find my way back to my goals? Reading my entries reminded me that though it would be exhausting at first, I could build back up again slowly. One sunny day two weeks later I walked for three hours.

All of us will have breaks in our routine. With commitment and determination, we can catch the curve balls life throws at us and toss them back again.

START JOURNALING

Go back and re-read your FIT Journal entries. Then make a list of the things that might interfere with your progress. Make another list of things you can do when that happens. Change your routine. Find the inspirational quotes that can become your mantra through tough times. Visualize your new body and the fun you'll have with it.

You're the best judge of what will work to re-energize and inspire you through setbacks.

Power Source Tool #9

Create Rewards and Celebrate Your Successes

"The road to success is always under construction."

–LILY TOMLIN

Everyone needs encouragement, and rewards are one of the best incentives to keep us motivated. Think of how much better children act when they know Santa Claus is coming. Think of the bonus systems that spark employees to reach extraordinary sales goals.

Why should it be any different for you and your fitness? You will be more successful in your fitness journey if you find ways to motivate and reward yourself. You deserve it.

The key is to find different ways to reinforce your fitness successes. These can range from complimenting yourself on your fitness efforts to making a pact with a partner to celebrate milestones along the way. The act of reinforcement itself is more important than the method.

Susan's Story

The marathons changed virtually every aspect of my life. I learned about passion, hard work, continuous improvement, discipline, focus, perseverance, and hands-on dedication.

I also learned to accept the limitations of my body and to celebrate every success, whether big or small.

I learned to be gentle with myself, to embrace nature and solitude, to relax, and to always stay focused on the present.

I took time to examine what I had learned, what worked, and what I might have done differently.

I now understand that, for me, speed doesn't matter as long as the determination and passion are there.

My rewards have included a healthy body, celebrating with family and friends, new clothes, facials, foot massages, and even fitness-focused trips.

Theresa's Story

One way I reward myself after a long run on a Saturday morning with my friend Peter or my YMCA friends is to get together afterwards for a morning beverage or a light breakfast and enjoy the company and conversation. It is such a rewarding feeling when you top off a good morning workout by celebrating with great friends.

The greatest reward I get from my running is a healthier and happier me. A healthy mind and body has always been a priority to me. Without it, my quality of life is diminished and I become susceptible to a host of problems that in turn affect my daily functioning and my ability to be the best I can be. As I said earlier, it is my survival tool.

When I teach a Cycle Fit class, the rewards are external. Hearing the participants say the class was great and that they got a good workout empowers me and makes me feel good. I like knowing that I am helping my Cycle Fit participants get the most out of their class so they can walk away and feel good about their fitness accomplishments.

SEVEN STRATEGIES FOR CREATING REWARDS AND CELEBRATING SUCCESSES

#1. Focus on self-improvement and don't compare yourself with others

While competition can be a great motivator, missing a goal can kill your momentum. Doing your best should never be viewed as a failure — even if someone else's best was better.

To stay motivated, you need to *recognize* your progress, not merely track it. Tracking is taking note of reaching a certain stage in your process. Recognizing involves taking the time to look at the bigger picture to realize exactly where you are and define how much you have left to do.

#2. Use music for motivation and reward

Music is a great tool in fitness; it can provide a tempo for your gym workouts and crank up your energy during runs and walks.

#3. Build on the momentum of your successes

This is one of the easiest and most powerful ways to stay motivated. As soon as you achieve one of your goals, take time to reward yourself in some way.

#4. Choose tangible ways to celebrate success and reward yourself

For some tasks, just taking a break and relaxing for a few minutes is enough. For others, you may want to give yourself a treat.

#5. Reward yourself on a continuing basis

Reward yourself for behavioral changes, such as breaking

habits and creating new routines, as well as for physical changes. The more you reward yourself for honestly made progress, the more motivated you will feel about reaching new milestones and, finally, accomplishing your goal.

#6. *Take time to look at the bigger picture*
As you begin to master ways to keep your motivation high, it will become easier for you to stay focused. You will have fewer moments of frustration and you'll find you actually achieve success and reach your targets faster. Reflect back on your biggest successes, achievements, and areas of progress.

#7. *Try some of these rewards and ways to celebrate, as suggested by our Power Source Women:*
- Take a long, relaxing bubble bath by candlelight.
- Buy a new book and schedule uninterrupted time to read it.
- Sign up for a team sport, such as baseball, basketball, or hockey.
- Rent a boat and spend the day soaking up sunshine with family and friends.
- Go to a concert or theatrical event you've been wanting to see.
- Buy some new workout music on iTunes.
- Purchase new cookware or other cooking gadgets.
- Upgrade your workout wardrobe.
- Sign up for dance lessons.
- Throw a dinner party, cook your favorite healthy foods, and celebrate with friends.
- Buy new lingerie.
- Book personal training sessions or Pilates sessions.

- Buy new exercise equipment.
- Purchase or make a special piece of jewellery: a bracelet, necklace, earrings, or rings. Every time you wear it, you'll be reminded of your successes.
- Begin a collection: stamps, thimbles, spoons, dolls, action figures, sports memorabilia, etc. Each time you achieve a goal, buy another item for your collection.
- Get a massage or a gift certificate for a massage when you achieve specific goals.
- Get your hair done. Try something daring.
- Get a makeover with a professional. And when you're all made up, get a glamor shot.
- Book a manicure and pedicure. Try a sparkling new color.
- Have a night out at the movies with a friend you haven't seen for a while.
- Attend an art show or visit a gallery or local museum.
- Go to your local amusement park and recapture the excitement you felt as a child.
- See your favorite sports team play live. Reward yourself with the best seats you can afford.

OUR POWER SOURCE EXPERT, RUTH KRONGOLD, SPEAKS

Success is definitely sweeter when I share it with my loved ones and friends. Celebration can be as simple as lingering over a good book in the morning sun with coffee in hand, resting bundled up in layers of down after a freezing swim, or lying on the dock in the summer heat after a long afternoon swim with head tingling and body air-drying as waves lap against the shore.

Success is also having the confidence to plan and make wonderful excursions to beautiful, sometimes remote, places.

Shared laughter comes easily in these sparkling moments of celebration.

OUR POWER SOURCE WOMEN SPEAK

We asked our Power Source Women for specifics on how they reward themselves and celebrate their successes.

Audrey

I just feel good about myself and appreciate my body for what it can do.

Edna

I assess my results by the number of people who tell me I inspire them and whether there are increased requests for my personal trainer services. I usually celebrate successes by joining a friend for a glass of wine.

Pat

After finishing my runs, I have coffee with friends and laugh. In terms of celebrating success, setting running goals provides the challenge for me and gives me immense satisfaction. I have trained for, and completed, two Ottawa Marathons and two half-marathons, plus numerous 5 and 10k runs.

I have also collected more than $25,000 for the Terry Fox Run over the years and have participated in every event to date (29 of them so far).

Phyllis

I love to hear feedback from my participants. Knowing they had a good workout inspires me to keep fine-tuning my classes.

OUR ROLE MODEL #5: SHEILA RHODES

MY STORY

It should not have happened to me. But it did.

I have always described myself as the poster girl for the Heart and Stroke Foundation in terms of how to live a healthy lifestyle. I have always been a very active person. I eat a low-fat vegetarian diet. I have never been overweight. I have never smoked. I exercise every day. There is no history of heart disease in my family. What more could a person do?

Six years ago I was out for my early morning 10k run as I had been doing every day for many years. After that would be a workout in the gym for at least an hour and a half, perhaps two hours. This was my normal routine. As I started my run, I noticed a slight discomfort in my chest. I thought I was getting a spring cold or maybe allergies. The discomfort continued for the next few weeks whenever I exercised.

Eventually I couldn't ignore it any longer. It was interfering with my sacred exercise routine. I reluctantly took myself to a walk-in clinic and described my symptoms. The doctor immediately sent me to the hospital where I underwent a full day of tests. I left with a prescription for an anti-inflammatory and was told to return if the pain did not go away in a few days.

Well, the pain did not go away. This led me to the cardiologist's office for a treadmill stress test. The results were not what I had expected. An angiogram was scheduled for the following Wednesday.

As I was lying in the recovery room after the test, the cardiologist appeared and told me I was not leaving the hospital until I had quadruple by-pass surgery. The surgery took place five days later. Two arteries had

90-percent blockage and another two were nearly as bad. Me — the picture of health. What a shock.

MY WAKE-UP CALL

As I was recovering in the hospital, one emotion was overwhelming. I was angry — very angry. I told every doctor who would listen that this should not have happened to me. I had done everything right.

Finally, one doctor put it in perspective when she calmly explained that if I had not led the exemplary lifestyle I was so proud of, I would have been dead at the age of 35.

I was 52 when this happened. Talk about a reality check.

MY SOLUTION

I am a very logical, scientific person and I needed answers. It didn't satisfy me to hear, "Sometimes we don't know why these things happen." I became an advocate for my own health.

On my follow-up visit six weeks after the surgery, the cardiologist suggested an additional blood test he was just hearing about. As it turned out, I had an elevated level of lipoprotein(a) — in fact, more than 12 times the normal level and five times over the level considered dangerous. It has the same effect as plaque on artery walls but was not detected in the cholesterol tests I had on a regular basis. It is a hereditary condition and had nothing to do with my lifestyle.

As a result, I was enrolled in a research project at McMaster Health Centre studying this condition. They were very interested in me.

MY FITNESS ROUTINE

My fitness routine fits my body rhythm. It starts at 4:30 a.m. I exercise 365 days a year, despite being told a day off is good for you. It just doesn't feel right if I don't exercise.

My morning run always begins the day no matter what the weather is like — I just wear different clothes if I have to. As a long-time member of the YMCA, I take advantage of Cycle Fit classes, weight training, water jogging, and yoga to balance my fitness activities. Being part of this community is a huge part of my life.

The following example demonstrates my passion for fitness. The day after my surgery, the physiotherapist came to get me up for a walk. He innocently brought a metal walker to my bedside. When he saw my running shoes under the bed, he quipped, "I guess maybe you don't want to use this."

According to the hospital's protocol, my fitness routine for the next 30 days was to increase my walking by one minute per day until I finally reached 30 minutes of exercise. Immediately on hearing this, I asked if I could do more. As soon as I returned home four days later, I was walking from 90 minutes to two hours at a time. My daily 10k runs began again six weeks after the surgery, only because the cardiologist pleaded with me to wait that long.

THE RESULT

The reason I am able to tell this story is that I took care of my health and did all the right things. It never occurred to me that one day my level of fitness would actually save my life.

It took a few months for that to really sink in and for me to accept that sometimes things do just happen.

WHAT I LEARNED

Looking back, I realize how fortunate I was to have grown up in a family in which physical activity and healthy eating were a given. We played outside every day until we were told to come in for dinner or it got too dark to see the skipping rope. That is not a reality for many children today, which should be a concern to you as a parent, grandparent, aunt, or sister.

The Heart and Stroke Foundation's 2010 Annual Report on Canadians' Health is titled *A Perfect Storm of Heart Disease Looming on our Horizon*. It warns that a perfect storm of risk factors and demographic changes are converging to create an unprecedented burden on

Canada's fragmented system of cardiovascular care, and no Canadian — young or old — will be left unaffected. Young people are beginning their adult lives with multiple risk factors for heart disease. Over the past 15 years, Canada has seen significant increases in overweight and obesity, high blood pressure, and diabetes. It used to be thought that, like heart disease and stroke, Type 2 diabetes and high blood pressure were diseases of aging. These increases will translate into an explosion of heart disease in the next generation.

PASSION TIPS FROM SHEILA RHODES

Be passionate about leading a healthy lifestyle and inspiring the next generation.

I am passionate about fitness and leading a healthy lifestyle, but I do not push my beliefs on other people — at least most of the time.

I teach a Health and Physical Education course to teacher candidates in a Faculty of Education. Several weeks into the course, I tell my personal story. Needless to say, the students are shocked. These young people are going into one of the best professions in the world and they need to be educated about the growing problem we have in Canada with childhood obesity and inactivity — two major causes of heart disease.

If I can inspire them to look at their own lifestyles and to remember how they are role models for their students, then I will have been successful as a teacher. I hope I have been a role model for these teacher candidates and that they will take my story with them long after they leave the faculty.

Read the latest research about heart disease and talk to your doctor. The leading causes of death among Canadian women are heart disease and stroke. It could happen to you. It happened to me, but I survived to tell my story.

Find an activity you enjoy and can do easily. Join a fitness center in your neighborhood because the friends you make there will keep you on track. Trust me, if you do not make it to the gym one day, your friends will expect a really good reason for your absence. That will keep you motivated and encouraged to come back again and again.

Buy a skipping rope and skip with your grandchildren. Take them for walks and to play tag in the park.

Volunteer to lead a yoga class in the local school.

Most of all, have fun.

JOURNALING WITH LESLEY SHORE

"The reward of a thing well done is to have done it."
–Ralph Waldo Emerson

Although I grew up in an era of relative prosperity, memories of the Great Depression were still a strong influence. Rewarding success was not the way we did things. I was expected to do well, and that was reward in itself (as Emerson expresses above). Times have changed and women have further changed them. But I still have trouble being kind to myself.

Now I'm contemplating the luxury of a mani-pedi as the reward for having got back on track after my recent bout of illness.

When I taught teachers, I suggested my students make lists of one-minute rewards they could squeeze into their packed teaching days, and another list of five-minute rewards.

A Starbuck's latte is a great reward on a morning when it's been hard slogging to get to your finish line. A trip to a yoga retreat somewhere warm and exotic might be your end-of-year celebration.

START JOURNALING

How comfortable are you in celebrating your own successes and rewarding yourself? Use your FIT Journal to make lists of your own. What are some very quick rewards that would please you? Which longer ones would you prefer? Is there something very special you would like to do to celebrate one year of being faithful to your new routines?

Power Source Tool #10

Assess Your Results and Set New Goals

"Without leaps of imagination, or dreaming,
we lose the excitement of possibilities.
Dreaming, after all, is a form of planning."

–GLORIA STEINEM

As with any other activity in your life, it's tempting to fall into a routine when it comes to fitness. That's actually all some people want: a routine that maintains their health. There's nothing wrong with that. There's no reason that everyone should be aiming to run marathons or take part in extreme fitness programs.

However, even the simple *maintenance* of fitness will require you to reassess your goals and activities and make adjustments. After all, ways of maintaining your fitness will change as you age.

Assessing your results and setting new goals is a good strategy to follow. It's important to look for ongoing improvement in your fitness program. It's the highs that will take you through the lows. It's the commitment to keep going that will make your journey a success.

Realize how fitness empowers you. Enjoy feeling more confidence, control, and motivation in maintaining your fitness and health once you start to see results than when you started your program.

Finally, with your newfound self-awareness, confidence, and self-esteem, set new goals for the future: short-term goals, long-term goals, and blue-sky goals.

Susan's Story

Through running marathons and half-marathons, I gained new respect for everyone who sets and achieves blue-sky goals. I know how tough it is to get the results you desire. In the end I learned that if you believe in yourself, anything is possible.

I now view myself as someone who has a healthy and fit body, and I am finally comfortable with my new weight and shape (which is 15 pounds more than I was in my 30s — and 20 pounds less than I was five years ago). And I have stopped weighing myself every day.

The changes have affected every aspect of my life. I now welcome structures, habits, and routines. I am more focused and less competitive.

After completing two marathons, I was excited to discover that I no longer felt as if I ever needed to do another. I knew I had achieved something remarkable — twice — and was comfortable with not wanting to commit the time and effort to train for yet another one. Instead, I am happy to complete half-marathons in three hours and to train for them by following my regular fitness routines.

I appreciate the fact that my current fitness program enables me to feel fit, control my weight, reduce stress, gain energy, and increase my self-esteem. Each year I do two or three half-marathons, which are easier to achieve and more enjoyable than a full one. In the future I plan to combine fitness with travel by signing up for these races in exotic places and planning some hiking and walking vacations.

And one day I'd like to get into yoga and get back into swimming.

Theresa's Story

I have developed a healthy, satisfying relationship with my fitness. My strongest connection has been with running. Running has sometimes been my source of power, giving me the capacity to free my mind from the day-to-day stresses with an uplifting impact on my mood.

Running has contributed to building my inner spirit. It has energized me and helped me appreciate my body's potential to move through many miles and many marathon celebrations.

I changed when I started to run. I became a stronger and happier woman. I found new friends and challenged my abilities. The reason I conquered many marathons was I began to believe in myself.

I cannot stress enough how critical physical fitness has been to my life. It is a key component, along with good mental fitness and optimal nutrition. I believe these three factors have contributed to my higher level of functioning and my ability to keep training. I believe my 19 marathons have been injury-free because I have listened to my body and allowed sufficient time for recovery and renewal when the time was right.

As I reflect on my ongoing passion for fitness and health through my running and teaching of Cycle Fit classes, I realize I still have many goals to reach: Learning to teach a Zumba® class, returning to judo, and beginning to cycle outdoors are today's physical fitness aspirations. I have a wonderful lifelong relationship with my fitness and I plan to make my journey exciting and rewarding along the way.

Perhaps one day I will move on from running marathons. If and when I do, I will never forget the power of the runners who believed in me. I will be eternally grateful to my many running friends and to the running groups I have had the good fortune to join.

SEVEN STRATEGIES FOR ASSESSING YOUR RESULTS AND SETTING NEW GOALS

#1. List the areas that challenged you and the lessons you learned
Take time to examine the ways you may have sabotaged your fitness program, the problems you have experienced, and how you can modify your expectations and your program in the future.

#2. Be proud of yourself
Identify your top fitness accomplishments and your successes: the races you entered, the laps you swam in the pool, the hikes you completed, or the people you inspired and coached through your own fitness program.

#3. Summarize the lessons in your FIT Journal
Have you:
- Directed some of your daily activities and actions toward achieving better fitness? Achieved a more balanced fitness program than you when you started?
- Noticed which fitness activities made you feel better, making them worth the time and work involved?
- Managed to stick to your scheduled workout or activity plan?
- Incorporated more variety into your fitness program and your diet?
- Gained an understanding of your patterns of activity and inactivity?
- Become aware of the importance of pursuing a balanced life?
- Experienced a fitness-related "rush" or exercise high?

- Learned to accept and be grateful for your body and to celebrate its ability to change?

When you find yourself facing an obstacle, take out your FIT Journal and read it.

#4. Register for a fitness-focused event or take a fitness-based vacation

Sign up for a 5k walk, a charity bike ride or run, a swim competition, a women's cycling weekend, a yoga retreat, or a hike in a national park.

Find a vacation destination where you can be active. Check out your hotel to see if a fitness center is available to guests or ask for suggested running and walking routes. Plan vacations where you can do a lot of walking. It's a great way to burn calories and see a city or town.

Take portable equipment on your next trip to use in your hotel room, such as resistance bands, skipping ropes, and tubing. Stability balls with pumps can be deflated and packed in your suitcase.

Sign on for a challenging fitness-focused green vacation, such as a yoga retreat or a hiking trip. **G**

Walk the beach instead of sunbathing. **G**

#5. Review the Green FIT tools we have incorporated in this book and develop your own Green FIT Action Plan.

Following are our suggestions.

Green FIT Action Plan

Sustaining our planet has become a mission for many of us. We are always looking for ways to decrease the negative impact our lifestyles can have on our environment.

There are so many different ways to increase natural energy through the decisions you make each day. For instance, by opening your curtains or window blinds and allowing the natural light to shine through, you eliminate the need for electricity. But that's just one example. There are other ways you can return to a natural way of living. Each chapter of *Power Source for Women* includes natural living tools and ideas that you can immediately incorporate into your daily life.

Right now, we want to focus on ways you can tap into saving our planet by incorporating green practices into your fitness plan or activities.

Take the following steps with our Green FIT Action Plan and start building a fitness routine that will help you understand and nurture your relationship with the natural world. This will help you become more connected with your community — and planet.

So let's get Green FIT!

Going green with your fitness workout and activities can be a great way to add zest to your relationship with fitness and food. Spend more time outdoors and you will suddenly begin to meet more of your neighbors and connect with nature. Enjoy the sounds and scents around you and appreciate where you are in the moment. Try taking a vacation from your conventional gym and go outdoors.

Ways to get into the Green FIT spirit include:

- gardening
- hiking
- walking
- golfing
- jogging
- mountain biking

- swimming
- roller blading
- skiing
- snowshoeing
- snowboarding
- shoveling snow

Find a Green Gym

Have you heard of the Green Gym program? Well if you haven't, you soon will. It started in Europe and is spreading around the world. It's an outdoor fitness movement that is lightly structured with a no-cost program consisting of groups of people who meet one to three times a week and get active, have fun, and do their part, together, for the preservation of our planet.

Activities include composting and reforestation efforts. Both are educational as well as physical, and both are excellent ways to conserve our planet.

The program starts by including a warm-up and a cool-down to get you prepared for green action. This is a positive way to connect with your community, build new relationships, get healthier, and contribute to the wellness of our world.

Look for green fitness groups in your community. If you can't find one, start one. What a great initiative to take: making your community greener through fitness.

Customize the program to your liking and to the environment you live in. Start connecting with like-minded people and get together to act for the good of your bodies and your world.

Four Green FIT Kitchen Exercises

Turn your kitchen tasks into an energizing eco-friendly experience and you may just begin to build a better relationship with those jobs that just have to be done.

1. *Dishwashing Stretch*: Ignore the dishwasher and begin dishwashing stretches before, during, and after you wash.

Start by loading the sink half-full with dishes and then fill the sink just above the dishes with *cool* water (remember we are saving energy). Now grab the edge of the counter in front of the sink — holding on tight — and, slowly stepping back, stretch out as far as you can go. Hold that position to the count of ten.

Return to an upright position and begin to wash your dishes.

Try to take periodic 10-second stretch breaks throughout the task. Do as many as you can until the dishes are clean.

At the end, finish up with a final stretch. Lower your head and breathe gently for 10 seconds.

It may take more time for you to wash the dishes, but just think of the benefits you will gain and the new connection with dishwashing that you will have.

2. *Eco-sweep*: Turn sweeping into an opportunity to practice your ballroom dancing.

To begin: Put away the vacuum for those dusty floors. Grab a tall broom and turn on the music. Start sweeping with your new dance partner, Mr. Broom. You'll have fun and get the endorphins pumping as you eco-sweep your way to cleaner floors.

3. *While You Wait Push-ups*: While waiting for the

kettle to boil or the coffee to brew, try doing some wall push-ups.

Stand in front of the wall far enough away so your fingertips can touch the surface.

Position your feet so they are stable and shoulder-width apart.

Now, lean forward so your palms are resting on the wall and your body is on a slight slant.

Inhale deeply and slowly exhale as you move your body toward the wall until your nose touches it.

Slowly breathe in as you begin to move your body back to your original position.

Try doing this five times and build up the repetitions as you get stronger. Feel free to cut the reps when the kettle is boiled or the coffee is brewed.

4. *Grocery Bag Lifts*: Each time you go shopping, be sure to take advantage of those heavy bags to do a little arm building.

When you get home from the grocery store with the bags, instead of unpacking, start lifting.

Lift a bag five times to the front, side, and rear. Try to complete up to three sets of five repetitions for each arm.

Once you've completed your kitchen grocery bag lift, you'll feel invigorated and ready to unpack.

#6. *Set new goals that are adventurous, ambitious, and blue-sky*

Here are some exciting fitness trends to get you started:

1. Zumba® classes. The Zumba® program fuses hypnotic Latin rhythms and easy-to-follow moves to create a one-of-a-kind fitness program. The routines feature interval-training sessions. Fast

and slow rhythms and resistance training are combined to tone and sculpt your body while burning fat.

2. Yoga fusion. This update on a classic can involve a blend of yoga, aerobic dance, cycling, boxing, or yoga and spinning.

3. JUKARI, Fit to Fly. In 2008 Reebok and Cirque du Soleil joined forces to shake up and invigorate women's gym routines. This is an hour-long total body workout using a FlySet that combines cardio, strength, balance, and core training.

4. Balancing technical precision with free-form expression, Nia brings the body, mind, emotions, and spirit to optimum health through music, movement, and self-expression.

5. Kettlebells. This is a popular Russian dumbbell workout. It may feel a bit like flinging a bowling ball around a room for 30 minutes, but advocates say it's an incredible fat-burning workout. A Kettlebell looks like a cannonball with a handle. Using them combines cardiovascular, muscle strength, muscle endurance, and flexibility training into a program that is efficient and complete.

6. Tabata, a four-minute workout. This high-intensity interval training was originally developed for Japan's Olympic speed-skating team. It has become a favorite high-speed workout.

7. Exciting new water exercise classes:
   • Water yoga. The buoyancy and hydrostatic pressure of water supports the body during traditional yoga poses in warm water.

- Ai Chi. Slow-flowing movement through warm water. Great for relaxation or stretching. Ai Chi is designed to strengthen and tone the body while also promoting relaxation and a healthy mind–body relationship. The technique was developed in Japan in the 1990s and is now practiced all over the world, particularly in North America.
- Aqua jog. This is a high-intensity, no-impact aerobic workout in deep water designed to increase aerobic fitness as well as tone and strengthen muscles.
- Arthritis aquatics. This type of class helps to improve joint flexibility and muscle strength.
- Water kickboxing. This is a low-impact, high-intensity aerobics program that incorporates kickboxing moves in the water.

8. Martial arts such as Kenpo increase muscle tone, flexibility, endurance, coordination, and speed. They create a feeling of focus in daily life, increased self-esteem, respect for self and others, and self-discipline.

9. Other new workout combinations include Disco Yoga (disco music and yoga), cycle karaoke (sing as you cycle), and HydroRide (spinning in the pool).

#7. Examine the strategies and tools offered in the chapters of this book and look at your areas of strength and improvement as you set goals for the future. What have you achieved in your life as a result of your fitness?
- Evaluate the type of fitness plan that works for you and create strategies to work around your biggest obstacles.

- Seek out information, guidance, or support related to getting in shape or taking your fitness program to a new level from books, magazines, websites, blogs, retail outlets, trainers, health professionals, and fit friends.
- Share your goals with other people, including your accountability team, and ask for their support.
- Experiment with different kinds of fitness routines or activities.
- Work out in a class or with a group.
- Become more interested in nutrition. Read and understand nutrition labels, articles, and websites.
- Review your FIT Journal and your Weekly FIT Training Log.
- Push yourself past what you think you can do.
- Spend more time being physically active with friends and family.
- Participate in athletic events or competitions.
- End the year feeling more hopeful and excited about your fitness commitment and program than when you started the year.

OUR POWER SOURCE EXPERT, RUTH KRONGOLD, SPEAKS

I know I'm doing well from a fitness perspective when I am energized by activity, sleep relatively peacefully, eat well, experience minimal pain, have a feeling of generosity that motivates my actions, and approach life with a sense of hope. I feel ready to carry the responsibilities of my work, enjoy time with friends and family, and am at peace when I am alone.

My basic daily swim is now 130 laps or 3.25 km. It would be conservative to say that I swim about 1000 km per year and have done so for more than three decades. The circumference of our earth is 40,075.02 km. It is my goal to "swim around the world" and reach the 40,075.02 km mark before I am 65 years old. That would be an exciting milestone for me. Around the world in 40 years. Maybe the moon, at a circumference of 10,921 km, will be my first objective.

OUR POWER SOURCE WOMEN SPEAK

We asked our Power Source Women to describe how they assess their results, what new fitness goals they have set, and what they have achieved in their lives through being fit.

Audrey

I like to try some new fitness activities every year. This takes me to places other than my own fitness club and allows me to meet active people and learn new things. My fitness dream is to still be doing this when I'm 80.

Edna

I am happy to continue to work out five times a week as well as with my personal training clients. I certainly do not want to overtax my body at this stage of my life, but I'm happy to keep challenging it.

Pat

My goals for the future are to be in shape, to maintain good health, and to stay injury free.

Phyllis

I am more aware of my body today than ever before. Although I would still like to lose some weight, I know what it takes to do that, so my plan is to focus on health. I still have the occasional trigger, but I have my exercise routine, which helps me tremendously as I strive toward increasing my fitness.

Also, I am trying to attend more classes from other fitness instructors. I have always avoided attending other classes, but that is slowly changing. I now recognize I can learn from others. I see the need to add this to my fitness program.

My goal for the future is to keep dancing, because I love to dance, and to develop more exciting and energetic classes for my students.

JOURNALING WITH LESLEY SHORE

"Amidst the worldly comings and goings, observe how endings become beginnings." –Tao Te Ching

The book you are holding in your hands may be coming to an end, but I'm just beginning to think where this fitness journey might take me. In the short time that I've maintained this routine, the results have become manifest in all parts of my life.

The sun was brilliant when I woke up this morning, but I decided to change my sheets and then take a quick peek at the computer. A friend had sent an e-mail about a book sale with books at only $1.99 each. The catalogue had hundreds of books that would have taken me hours to scroll through.

I resisted. I slipped into my clothes and headed out the door for my walk in the ravine.

I've spent the rest of the day working in the kitchen because company is coming for dinner. I can imagine how resentful I would have been feeling had I not gone for that walk this morning. Discipline is my weakness. I've made progress.

As ridiculous as a salsa class once seemed to me, I now admit that, someday, it may actually be a possibility.

Dreams achieved beget new dreams.

START JOURNALING

A fitter body equals a more disciplined mind, a richer soul, enhanced self-esteem, and the feeling you just might be able to accomplish anything you set your mind to do.

Look back on what you have achieved already. Read the pages of your FIT Journal.

Remember where your stumbling blocks were and how you worked around them. Write about how you are feeling now about your body and your life.

Where are you headed from here? What doesn't seem as impossible as it once did? Revise your fitness plan. Whatever you decide from here, aim high. You can do it.

Acknowledgments

Theresa and Susan's Acknowledgments:

Our thanks to our publisher, Don Bastian, and our web designer, Richard Hicken, both of BPS Books, and to our photographer, Shahrokh Saeedi.

Our thanks as well to:

The women who so generously shared their time, talents, and stories for our book: Ruth Krongold, Lesley Shore, Claire Vandramini, Maureen Catania, Abbey Smith, Gloria Jacobs, Sheila Rhodes, Audrey Korey, Edna Levitt, Pat McMonagle, Phyllis Naken, Monika Klein, Nadine Cowan, and Dorina Vendramin.

The women who encouraged us to create this book: Jane Claire Purden, Carol Washburn, Georgia Jacobs, Stephanie Warren, Mimi Donaldson, Tanya Craan, Loriana Sacilotto, Ellen Alban, Livia Grujich, and Cynthia O'Neill.

Active Adult magazine, for the profile and photos of Maureen Catania (January/February 2010).

Devon Blaine from the Blaine Group, for your professionalism and enthusiasm in designing and implementing an outstanding publicity campaign.

You our readers — we hope this book will be a constant resource to you, and we welcome your comments, suggestions, and additions.

Susan's Acknowledgments:

First of all, I'd like to thank Theresa Dugwell for collaborating on this book with me. It has been a labor of love and such a pleasure working with you.

My thanks also to my family: to my father, Harry Sommers, who taught and inspired me to exercise; to my husband, Peter, for his encouragement and commitment; to my two daughters, Andrea and Danielle, and their husbands, Eric and Allan; to my brother, Howard; and to my step-daughter, Kellie Keyes, and my new son-in-law, Danny Keyes.

I am especially grateful to Dr. Marla Shapiro, my doctor, role model, and friend for the past 30 years, for inspiring me to embrace a fit and healthy lifestyle.

Thanks to my coaches — Bev Tyler and Chen Cohen — for believing that I *could* do marathons even when I didn't! Thanks to the Running Room, where I have inspired others as a speaker and been inspired in their clinics. Also, to the instructors of my weights and spinning classes — Scott, Lily, and Lisa — for challenging me on an ongoing basis. Thanks to Sid Finkelstein for encouraging me to take my first Run Fit class in 2002 and for cheering me on ever since.

And my thanks to all of the women who are at the YMCA at 6 each morning with me — including Maxine, Rochelle, Mary, Peggy, Ellie, Frances, Gloria, Kum, Toni, and Carol — for making sure I'm there and giving me a hard time when I'm not.

A special thank-you to the wonderful people I have worked with at the Alzheimer Society of Toronto over the past three years and to Jane O'Hare for believing in me.

Thanks to my grandchildren — Lauren, Jonah, Seth, Dylan, Emily, and Molly — for teaching me what it means to be passionate, playful, and grateful for life!

Finally, thanks to all of my friends and family who have supported me and encouraged me throughout my life.

Theresa's Acknowledgments:

Let me begin by thanking a very important lady who came into my life: my co-author Susan Sommers. It has been an enlightening and gratifying experience working with you in creating this book. Together we can help change the world by strengthening women.

Thank you, Don Maxwell, for being my intellectual guide and partner, and for being a creative contributor to this book. You introduced me to a field that has captured my attention for life — a deep debt of gratitude will always remain in my heart for you. Much of what I have learned over the past several years through my academic studies and my work within the field of psychology and psychophysiology has influenced me to strive for a stronger presence in this field as I map out my plans to earn my PhD.

I am grateful to:

My sisters, Cindy Roman and Kelly Dugwell-Bow, for being in my life and for the cherished moments when we can spend time together outside our busy lives. My niece, Brianna Clement: you are my brightest light and add sunshine to every day. My brother-in-law, Cesar Roman — thank you for inspiring my sister to find her fitness — and four special guys, Raymond Clement, Jim Bow, and my nephews James Bow and Brandon Roman. Kyla Maxwell-Jones: you are new to this world, but your tiny presence has already generated enormous love in many hearts.

I am also grateful to my friends: Alfred Carr, thank you for always believing that I had the potential to be so much more — I am fortunate to have you in my world; Melanie Straus, for your inspiration and support and for always finding beautiful ways to show you were thinking of me — may this book and our friendship inspire you to continue in your creation of your movie *Footprint*; Peter Tsekouras, for all the great conversations during those long runs while training for our marathons — you are one of the most positive, open-minded people I know and you are a great listener who always knows just what to say … it is such a pleasure running with you and I look forward to our next marathon; Al Cox, for your words of wisdom and your friendship along the way.

I also want to thank Chris Healy, my talented acting teacher: you taught me what it means to get out of my head and to never give up; Errol Lee, for your friendship and for bringing your beautiful music into my life and teaching me through your magical performances how "HEROS" are created; and my friend Michael Burgess, whom I so admire: you are truly a man who gives from the heart to so many charitable causes — through your music you have changed lives.

My thanks to my knowledgeable friend and alternative health-care practitioner, George Keramaris: you have the gift to heal; thank you for what you have taught me.

Normand Haas, thank you for continuing to encourage me to go for it in preparing for the Boston Marathon: you gave me a book once called *Ultra Marathon Man*, inscribed with a message that will always remain with me — "So many years of training … Hope this book gives you 90% inspiration instead of perspiration. Go for it, girl!"

Mary O'Regan, thank you for showing such enthusiasm and trying to find ways to connect me with like-minded women during the final stages of writing this book.

A special thank-you to: my friend Ryan Guthrie, for always cheering me on as I was writing this book and always offering me important tips to guide me on my journey; Maurice Cohen, for your strong words of encouragement and friendship; Ellen Alban, for the sunshine that you bring to our YMCA … your poetry represents your beauty inside and out; Gloria Weintraub, for your ability to always find the spirit from within to brighten any room — you made me smile many mornings; Nadine Cowan, you are a talented, energetic woman with enthusiasm to add value to many lives through your fitness training and vision of the future … I am grateful to have met you.

Sid Finkelstein, my journey of volunteering at the YMCA began because of you. You guided me and had faith in me and supported me as I became a leader … thank you.

Deidre Newman, thank you for making our multiple-marathon experience exhilarating and fun. We have celebrated many miles together.

Connie Chiang, you have taught me how to think outside the box when it comes to fitness.

Debbie Augustt-Moffatt and Maritza Requena Lupovici — my most enthusiastic and supportive cheerleaders — thank you for your friendship.

Michael Carter, thank you for always recognizing and appreciating my volunteer contribution to the Y. You were a bright light at the North York YMCA.

My thanks also to the YMCA of GTA, an amazing organization in Toronto to whom I now dedicate a part of my life. It is through encouragement, support, and friendships that I have gained and grown as a person. I will continue to spread the YMCA message to others who wish to develop as individuals and to create a greater sense of community and spirit.

Thank you to all my YMCA friends at the many locations throughout Greater Toronto, and especially: my North York YMCA friends, the YMCA Northern Backwards Running Group, whom I cherish as my lifelong friends; the many dedicated volunteers and the outstanding staff and general manager Jorge Rojas; and the Rocky Road Runners, for the incredible energy you bring to the world of running — your welcoming spirit has always made me feel a connection with your team.

May this book be a source of inspiration and motivation to the following special ladies as each of you strive to build a rewarding life-long relationship with your fitness and your health: Catherine, Anne, Mary, Laurel, Kathy, Sheryl, Daniela, Sophie, Tammy, and Sandra.

And finally to a special lady, Joyce Meyers, spiritual speaker and author: thank you for teaching my mother that there is hope for healing and to never give up.

About the Authors

SUSAN SOMMERS

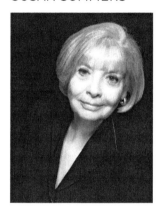

Born in New Jersey, Susan Sommers is one of Canada's most accomplished authors and experts in marketing and media relations. She established her own communication company in 1982 (Susan Sommers + Associates), has lectured in universities and at conferences across Canada, and has written four books on marketing and media relations.

Susan's vision of physical and mental fitness emerged from her own long-standing issues with weight and body image. She thus brings unique personal inspiration to her quest to mentor and educate women about the life-changing impact of a proper program of personal fitness. She has learned from her own inadequate strategies for dealing with physical challenges, including spending years at gyms without a "fitness for life" vision of higher-level conditioning.

Susan's perspective took a fundamental turn in 2002 when, at the age of 58, she began to walk and jog as a new Toronto YMCA member. From 2004 to 2007 she lifted weights and took aerobics classes, but more importantly she started training and signing up for races. Within three years she had completed a number of half-marathons and 10k and 5k runs. She won a medal for winning in her age category in a 5k run in Toronto in 2004. From 2004 to 2010, Susan completed 25 races, ranging from 5k to 42k.

These experiences were powerful motivators. Susan was further driven by the sight of her mother losing mobility due to osteoarthritis and Alzheimer's disease. Susan set a major challenge for herself: to complete the Scotiabank Toronto Waterfront Marathon in 2005, at the age of 61. Training for that marathon created the exhilaration of pushing hard toward a goal. Two years later, she accomplished the same feat again — completing the Scotiabank Marathon in a grueling seven and a half hours. She now combines her own marathon training with different levels of cross-training and appreciates her husband Peter's passion for running. He is a two-time Boston Marathoner, at ages 60 and 62.

A dynamic speaker, Susan has delivered motivational workshops related to fitness for women throughout North America. She is appreciated for her inspirational keynotes and seminars delivered to clients like LuluLemon Athletica, as well as Running Room retail outlets, fitness retreats, and conferences for Parks and Recreation. Susan is a strong contributing volunteer at the North York YMCA. She has served as public relations coordinator for the Breakfast of Champions and was the inaugural speaker for the YMCA Women's Speaker Series on defining achievement in personal fitness.

Susan is the mother of two daughters and a grandmother with six grandchildren.

THERESA DUGWELL

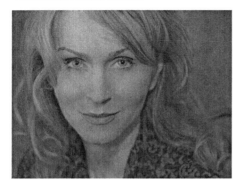

Theresa Dugwell operates PsyMetrics Professional Services, a Toronto-based company that offers psychological assessment services. She is a member of the Canadian Psychological Association, the American Psychological Association, and the Association for Applied Psychophysiology and Biofeedback.

Theresa is keenly aware of the importance of training the mind as well as the body. She works in the area of applied psychology, using biofeedback and neurofeedback modalities to help people build mental resilience through better regulation of the stress response.

Theresa believes that physical training is an integral part of optimal mind–body integration. Her own personal fitness program is rigorous and evolving and includes 19 completed marathons and several half marathons in the last 18 years. As part of her commitment to comprehensive health and wellness education, she mentors individuals to achieve a healthy lifestyle through mind–body fitness. She is a member of the Canadian Fitness Professionals Association and is a certified Lifeskills Coach and Facilitator, a Certified Spinning and Pilates Instructor, and a Fitness Instructor Specialist.

With an award-winning role in the volunteer program at Canada's largest YMCA, Theresa has produced the Breakfast of Champions and is a founding member of the North York YMCA Women's Fund, a program that assists women who are survivors of violence and abuse. This program provides YMCA memberships to women during critical life transitions, giving them access to a place of community, health, and support for personal growth.

As part of her inclusive and eclectic perspective on fitness, Theresa has given workshops on Emotional Intelligence in the Workplace, Creativity and Self-Esteem, Running for Beginners, and the Psychophysiology of the Stress Response. In addition she is Associate Producer of the Canadian feature film *Blueprint*. This film is a deep and honest study of one woman's struggle with depression, a woman who through fitness, friendship, and faith finds greater self-awareness, self-esteem, and self-acceptance.

About the Contributors

Emotional Fitness Expert and Coach Ruth Krongold, 59

Born and raised in Toronto, Ruth completed her master's degree in Social Work and went on to train in family mediation, mindfulness-based meditation, and narrative therapy. She is a member of the Ontario Association of Social Workers, the Ontario College of Social Workers and Social Service Workers, the Women's Counselling Referral and Education Centre, and the Narrative Community of Toronto.

Aware of the needs of women and children fleeing domestic violence for a safe and supportive community, Ruth is a founding member of the North York YMCA Women's Fund, which provides this disenfranchised group with resources for subsidized membership.

Working in the cancer community as a facilitator, psychotherapist, and volunteer has given Ruth the opportunity to help marginalized people find their own voices and choose actions based on their personal values. She is an ongoing supporter of and participant in the annual

Light the Night Walk, a community-based fundraiser for the Leukemia and Lymphoma Society of Canada.

Ruth lives in Toronto with her two university-aged "children" who bring love and challenge into her life every day.

Journaling Expert Lesley Z. Shore, 63

Dr. Lesley Z. Shore (EdD – OISE/UT) was Assistant Professor in the Department of Curriculum, Teaching, and Learning, responsible for Intermediate/Secondary English, at the Ontario Institute for Studies in Education (OISE), University of Toronto.

In her course Anne Frank and the Writing of the Adolescent Self, Lesley honored the importance of journal writing in the development of identity. Writers and writing are her passion. Lesley has taught from kindergarten to grade 12 in public, private, and Jewish schools in Ontario.

Her work has been published in a number of publications and academic journals. These articles include "'A Thousand Obligations': Anne Frank, Holocaust Education and Anti-Semitism in Changing Times"; "Self-Writing, Sex-Ed and the Creation of Adolescent Identity"; "'I Kept My Mouth Shut': Anne Frank on Sexuality and the Body"; "Sound Bites from Anne Frank"; "Good/Bad Girls and the Women Who Teach Them: A Renewed Call for Media Literacy"; and "Girls Learning, Women Teaching: Dancing to Different Drummers."

Lesley has been journaling since she was 14 years old.

OUR POWER SOURCE WOMEN

Audrey Korey, 62

Although Audrey is now addicted to fitness classes, she did not step foot inside a gym until she was 40. Growing up, Audrey hiked, skied, and played tennis with her family but never worked out. Today she is at group fitness classes five to six days a week. Her fitness activities include kickboxing, step, spinning, body sculpting, and interval training.

Edna Levitt, 70

Edna was trained and certified by the Certified Professional Trainers Network in Toronto in 2006. That year she launched her own business, 50+ Fitness, to focus exclusively on personal training for muscle toning, strength building, and enhanced physical performance for people in her own over-50 age group. Her strength-training practice includes instructing group fitness classes and working with clients one-on-one. Several of her clients are in their 80s. She also presents her Muscles Matter workshop to various women's groups.

Pat McMonagle, 61

Pat works out at a gym five days a week. She has curled since 1976, currently doing so twice a week at Toronto's Leaside Curling Club.

Pat started running in 1980 and completed her first 5k run in London, Ontario, that year. Since then she has participated in numerous runs, including marathons and half-marathons.

Phyllis Naken, 63

Phyllis created Dancercise in the late 1970s to combine her two loves: dance and exercise. She taught at various health clubs and community centers in her area. for 15 years before retiring to pursue a career in real estate, but continued to maintain her healthy lifestyle, working out five days a week. She returned to the dance floor in June 2009 and is currently teaching Dancercise classes.

Monika Klein, 53

Monika Klein, BS, CN, has nearly 20 years of experience in clinical practice offering her own unique health counseling skills and experience. She is the president of Coaching for Health, LLC, a California-based company devoted to health and wellness. Her company offers specialized weight and wellness programs. She is a clinical nutritionist, author, lifestyle coach, teacher, and health and wellness spokesperson.

Monika counsels in the areas of diet and nutrition, lifestyle, healthy exercise, nutrient supplementation, and stress management, including quality sleep.

She is also the past Southern California Education Chair for the International and American Associations of Clinical Nutritionists (IAACN).

Index

personal training, 63, 66–67, 79, 102, 105, 158, 179

Pilates, 1, 36, 37, 58, 60, 82, 107, 109, 158

Ramsay, Agnes (personal trainer), 71–72

Reno, Tosca (author), 72

Robbins, John (author), 46

Rock Band, 48

Self-Directed Soloist, 105, 106, 109, 115

S.M.A.R.T. goals, 77

Spirited Planner, 107, 108, 109, 117

Tabata, 176

triathlons, 11, 41, 78

trigger foods, 70, 71, 86, 93, 180

Vision Boards, 141–42

visualization exercises, 98, 110, 111–14

water kickboxing, 177

water yoga, 176

Weekly FIT Training Log, 65, 78, 109, 119, 127, 128, 130–33, 178

Wii Fit, 47

Wii Sports, 47

Wii video games, 47

YMCA, xiv, xvi, xvii, xviii, 9, 28-29, 37, 38, 39, 40, 41, 63, 64, 69, 156, 162

yoga, 1, 2, 12, 15, 33, 34, 37, 42, 47, 48, 60, 65, 80, 81, 92, 104, 106, 108, 109, 115, 117, 118, 163, 165, 168, 171, 176

yoga fusion, 176